# FAMILY HEALTH
*Care and Management at Home*

# FAMILY HEALTH

## *Care and Management at Home*

DR. ROBERT ANDREWS AND DR. KIRK HARGRAVE
*Illustrations by* RAY BURROWS

Pelham Books

First published in Great Britain by Pelham Books Ltd
52 Bedford Square, London WC1B 3EF
1976



ISBN 0 7207 0889 3

Set and printed in Great Britain by
A. Wheaton & Company, Exeter

# *Contents*

# *List of Illustrations*

Dedicated to the memory of
the late Dr Stephen Coulsdon Wake
beloved family doctor, Bideford, North Devon, 1931 - 73

# Introduction

With the upsurge in community medicines, and the fact that the most expensive medical treatment you can give to any patient is to put him into hospital, more and more conditions are being treated at home by the family (or community) doctor. Many conditions, like coronary thrombosis, are probably better treated at home than in hospital. There are an increasing number of old people in our population who need nursing care and attention as their health deteriorates.

This book sets out to give the fundamentals of home nursing, details of preparing a sickroom, and some information about special nursing conditions.

# 1
# *The nursing of children*

The nursing of the sick child nowadays is almost an anomaly. It is much more the management of sick children that is called for, and this will be gone into in detail in later chapters. The general principles for looking after a sick child are:

1. They should be confined to a room at even temperature.
2. If there is no specific reason for them to stay in bed, they can be up in the room, but they must not go out of the room, and certainly not outside.
3. When possible, toilet and washing facilities should be available on the same floor, and when the disease is infectious and there is some degree of isolation, a commode in the sick-room is very useful.
4. The room must not be too hot or too dry. Central heating, gas, electric fires, etc., take the moisture out of the air. Children with chest infections especially need moist air, and this can be achieved by boiling some water and allowing it to give off steam into the room. An electric kettle, if supervised, will do.
5. Whatever other care the sick child may require in its management, there is very little to beat tender, loving care.

Television is a great boon to the sick child and there is seldom a reason why he should not be allowed to see it. It is important that he be a part of the household as much as possible as the bored, unoccupied child takes much longer to get better than the interested, active child.

2

# Problems in child management

Coughs, colds, colics and fevers, and how to deal with them are perhaps the major home nursing problems for parents with young families. There are simple guide lines to be followed in these situations. There always comes the point, which is so difficult to decide, as to when, or when not, to send for the doctor, what to do if your child has a temperature, and the debatable question, when, or when not, to send your child to school.

### *When your baby has a cold*

A cold is, next to teething and feeding problems, perhaps the most common and disturbing crisis in baby management, for the baby with a cold will not only be miserable and fuss, but will probably go off his food, and not sleep. He may run a temperature, and it is possible that the combined set of circumstances will change the nature of his motions. As it progresses he will cough and may vomit stringy stuff. At this the worried mum, particularly if it is her first baby, may be at her wit's end. What can she do?

Of course it is wise to try to stop the set of circumstances arising by keeping a baby away from infection as far as possible. The common cold is a virus and is infectious, and if auntie who has a cold insists on cuddling the baby, he is far more likely to catch one than if you suggest she doesn't touch him. Anyone with a cold should keep away from a baby if possible; otherwise, it is a good idea to wear a mask or hold a clean handkerchief over your nose and mouth when going into the same room as a baby.

You cannot keep a baby away from people with colds

completely, but you can take the more obvious steps to keep him away from sources of infection. If he does catch a cold, remember that he is now a source of infection himself, and it's not the best time to take him to visit the baby next door.

Life, both on the TV and in baby's pram, is a continual battle between the goodies and the baddies, with the tide of battle swinging to and fro. So a second line of precaution is to get your baby's defences organised against germs and viruses. How can you do this?

The main defences are a good adequate diet with added vitamin supplements, and a sensible, practical routine. A fit, thriving baby will look after himself.

Make sure that your baby has plenty of fresh air and sunshine when available, as sunshine is a good source of vitamin D. Ensure he has adequate clothing—not too much or too little. If you put ten jumpers and five blankets on a baby you are just as likely to get him into trouble as you would if you left him in his vest in a snowstorm. Make sure that no clothing is too tight round the chest, as this can limit the amount a baby can expand his chest and will restrict his breathing.

When in the house try as far as possible to keep the room the baby is in at an even temperature. When you put him to bed, try to ensure there is not a great temperature drop in the room he is going to. It is asking for trouble to roast him in front of the fire for a couple of hours on a cold day, then put him into a cold cot in an ice-box of a bedroom.

If you are going out, wrap him up in the same way as you wrap up yourself, and tackle the elements heartily together.

It is important to see that a baby has adequate rest, for to be healthy he must have his full complement of sleep. If he is not sleeping at night as he should, see whether you are giving him too much or too little sleep in the afternoon, or if you are overtiring him so much that he is agitated and cannot sleep. Well rested, properly fed, and adequately clothed, he is well prepared to battle against germs.

If, in spite of all this, your baby does catch cold—and if he lives in this country he will be unique if he doesn't—what can you do about it? You will already know how it is going to affect him, so you aren't going to be too upset. Babies know when their mothers are upset and worried, and if you can hide your concern you are helping him already.

The cold will last several days. It is a virus infection, and no wonder-drug will kill off the germs during the first twenty-four hours. It has got to run its course. While it does, keep the baby's nose as clear as possible. If it is blocked his breathing is more difficult, and feeding, particularly bottle-feeding, becomes a fight both for you to get the milk down and for baby to get any breath while the milk is going down. Gently clean out both nostrils with cotton wool before each feed and see that the nasal airways are clear.

Your doctor can prescribe nasal decongestive drops suitable for a baby which can be of great help. Don't put any oily drops down, as these will only cause further clogging. Repeat the cleaning of the nostrils before you put him to sleep. Your baby will obviously sleep and take his food better if he can breathe through his nose.

Compromise on his feeding. Don't stick to normal routines but give him what he will take most easily. He will probably be inclined to take fluids rather than solids. Don't overtire him trying to force food down when he just doesn't feel like it—he will be better in a few days. Give him extra fluid if possible, as he is likely to get hot and perspire, increasing his liquid requirements.

Expect him to be sick occasionally. He cannot yet cough up mucus and tends to swallow it, and as he vomits it up from his stomach he will squeeze it out of his nose, chest and everywhere else and will be much better and clearer after he has done it.

A simple cough linctus will soothe an irritant cough that is keeping him awake and depriving him of his rest. Be sure to get the linctus specially prescribed for a baby from your doctor, and make sure you give only the quantity required for the baby's age. Don't, whatever you do, give the baby grandpa's cough mixture that you found in the bathroom cupboard—this could well do him harm.

If the baby's cold does not progress as you think it should, or is complicated by something like excess vomiting, obtain expert advice from the district nurse, health visitor, or doctor.

Expect, and arrange, to give more time to the baby for a few days. A mother's comfort and cuddling is an irreplaceable medicine. The baby will soon get over a cold and in doing so will have built up some resistance of his own against further colds.

If you have looked round any crowded room, be it filled with mini-skirted teenagers or doddering greybeards, you can be sure that all of them without exception will have had colds as babies and recovered and been none the worse for them in the long run, and so, certainly, will your baby. There is no need for you to worry.

*Coping with colic*

The two most common causes of pain and discomfort in small babies are teething and colic. It is not always possible to decide which is causing the trouble, but as a rule colic is associated with distensions and hardness of the abdomen; the pain comes in spasms and very often the baby will draw up his knees.

With teething there is the same amount of discomfort and distress, but rarely abdominal symptoms, and there are usually more direct signs such as red cheeks, excessive salivation, and a constant effort by the baby to relieve his discomfort by biting.

Before deciding that a baby's discomfort is more likely to be colic than teething, look for other causes such as a discharging ear, over-heating, or even some obvious discomfort like an open nappy pin.

If you decide that colic is really the cause of the baby's distress, what can be done to help? Bringing up the wind with the help of antacids gives some relief, but most important, of course, is to try to prevent the colic arising.

By far the biggest direct or indirect cause of colic is feeding. The position in which a baby is held while being fed is important. He is much more likely to take in air if he is lying down than if he is upright, so if he has a tendency to colic try feeding him in a rather more upright position.

Don't let him cry too much before a feed as he will be filled up with air, and tired before he starts. Comfort him and let him settle down happily as much as possible before the feed starts.

If a baby gulps his feed down too quickly while being breast-fed, his stomach will be blown up. This can be avoided if greater care is taken over feeding technique. Don't let the baby go at the breast too fiercely, particularly if there is an over-abundant milk supply; it may sometimes help to express a small amount of milk before he starts feeding. Try to make sure the feed is not over too quickly.

Colic is more common in bottle-fed babies. It is most important to find a teat with a hole just big enough to give controlled feeding. If the hole is too big the baby will gulp down large quantities of milk and air at the same time. If it is too small, he will have to suck so hard that half the time he will be taking in more air than milk.

It is essential to achieve an even flow and if you are unable to manage it properly yourself, do take advice from your midwife or health visitor.

When the baby starts on mixed feeding, too sudden a change or too much variety of type of food can lead to severe colic and bowel upset. To begin with, only one feed in the day should have the addition of solids and semi-solids, and the baby should have little more than a taste of whichever cereal you give first, made as a very dilute solution. If there is no colic or tummy upset, you can gradually increase the amount of food or the types of food you are offering. If the baby tolerates it all well, you can cautiously increase both the amount and variety.

The phenomenon known as three-month colic has never been satisfactorily explained, but many babies up to the age of three months scream for a period of about four hours a day with signs of colic, which tends not to be relieved by feeding or by the bringing up of wind. The trouble usually passes after the third month. Again it is important not just to assume that a baby has got colic, but to look out for any other causes.

If, however, nothing helps and the baby is going to scream

for a four-hour stretch a day, you can often arrange feeding and bathing times so that his screaming time is during the day, when only his rest is interrupted.

Strangely, this daily time of crying is most often between six and ten in the evening. This is more desirable from your point of view than if it is two to six in the morning. Do be prepared during this spell of three-month colic to give the baby some extra comforting. Unfortunately there is no magic pill to make a baby's colic vanish. Take comfort from the fact that the colicky baby is usually a thriving one and his troubles are a nuisance rather than serious. However, when a baby has persistent colic and is also listless and not thriving, then further help and medical investigation is required.

Many mothers wonder about the use of pacifiers. They range from the old-fashioned dummy to various new patent teats that hold small quantities of orange juice.

In principle, one should avoid the frequent use of a pacifier. There is some indication that it can lead to malformation of mouth and dental structure as well as being a possible source of infection.

Practically, if your baby's colic is keeping you and him awake and disturbing the household, and you have tried everything else but the only thing that will comfort him is a pacifier, then there is justification in using it.

But do remember a pacifier should be one of the last things one tries in the treatment of colic in the small baby.

### *When to treat a fever and when to leave it alone*

A fever in a child probably causes more unnecessary general alarm than any other single medical symptom; many families gear their activities to thermometer readings, rush into action with aspirin, ice cubes, and wet towels at the slightest rise in temperature. Often I will get a call—would I come and see John Smith, etc., he has a temperature. If it is a direct call, I can discuss the position with the parent and decide on the merits of the call, but if it is a second-hand message given by a neighbour, I have little alternative but to make a visit which frequently is unnecessary.

The most important step in assessing any illness is to add up the sum total of the symptoms, temperature or fever being only one of them. This is illustrated most clearly in a common condition like acute appendicitis, which it is possible to have without having any temperature rise. Most commonly there is a temperature rise in this condition, but it is usually in the region of 99°F. (37.3°C.) to 100°F. (37.8°C.). On the other hand, a very trivial condition can be associated with an extremely high temperature rise, say of up to 105°F. (39.5°C.).

Most people are happy to accept that a raised temperature is a danger signal and are foolishly reassured by a normal temperature as a sign that all is well. Most normal thermometers cannot read the lower temperature ranges and hypothermia, a serious condition in babies, would be missed if the ordinary household thermometer were used to assess their condition.

*What is a fever?* A fever exists when the body temperature goes above the normal body range of 95°F. (35°C.) to 99°F. (37.3°C.). Fever is a symptom alone, not a condition in itself, and it is an indication that the body is trying to resist an infection. A fever is, in fact, part of our defence mechanism against disease. It attacks the invading organisms in the following ways:

1. A high temperature often limits the growth of many viruses. It also produces a specific substance in the body that is thought to be the first line of defence against many common viral infections.
2. A raised temperature helps mobilise white blood cells which combat bacterial infections, acting in a similar way to putting a poultice on a local infection like a boil, stimulating the white blood cells to move to the area, encourage the blood flow to the area and rid the body of infection. Once the white cells are increased in number, this is a factor in lowering the fever.
3. Fever also stimulates certain of the ductless glands to produce enzymes which help in the body's defence mechanism against infection.

*When to treat a fever* When to treat a fever is often a difficult decision. The important thing is to treat the complaints of the child with a fever.

The first step in the presence of fever and the general malaise that is associated with it, i.e. flushed face, rapid pulse, loss of appetite, thirst, aching limbs, etc., is to check your child, by questions when possible, and by examination, to see if there is a single presenting cause.

1. Are the eyes red and congested?
2. The throat. Is it sore to swallow? If you can get a look at the back of the throat, are the tonsils enlarged?
3. The ears. Do they hurt? Are they discharging?
4. The neck. Is it stiff? Are the glands obvious?
5. The chest. Is there a cough? Is there any particular part of the chest that hurts more than the rest?
6. The stomach. Does it hurt anywhere? Does the child feel sick?
7. The limbs. Apart from generalised ache, does one part hurt more than the rest?
8. Is there a sign of infection anywhere, such as a septic finger, boil or raised red lumps?
9. Is there a rash anywhere on the body?

Often a visit to a child with a fever requires no more than the bedclothes being turned back to show one of the common infectious diseases like chicken pox, the mother having been so concerned about the temperature rise she did not bother to look any further.

If you do feel you need a visit from the doctor in the circumstances where your child has a fever, do collect as much information as possible before you send for him as it helps him to decide:

1. If there is any need to come.
2. The degree of urgency of the visit.
3. Whether he should bring some particular medicine with him.

If a child presents as being hot, with no other complaint than the normal discomfort associated with being hot, then generally you can treat the local discomfort and see what happens. In so many cases the child will have thrown off whatever was attacking it by the next day.

There is usually a demand for an increase in fluid intake, and this is always important. The single danger from fever on its own is dehydration. It can give rise to all sorts of problems, particularly in the balance of blood chemistry, if it is not corrected with adequate fluids.

Do not give aspirin as a routine. It has a part to play but has some dangers of its own. If you feel you have to give aspirin, then it is better to use the soluble type for children, and important not to exceed the dose recommended by the manufacturer. Give it only for specific symptoms such as headache or limb ache.

When a child has a previous history of convulsions in the presence of a high temperature, cooling the child by tepid sponging does reduce the risk of further convulsions.

A fever that is not settling after 24-48 hours, where the child is obviously not so well, is an indication that medical advice should be sought.

An American doctor once said, "I try to get mothers to recognise that fever is not a horrible enemy one must fight but, in fact, is your friend combating whatever infection the child has". To me fever is like the alarm at a fire station. It tells us when there is a fire (infection) but not how serious a fire (infection), and the parent whose main concern is how to lower the fever is like a fireman who worries over turning off the alarm but forgets the fire that caused it.

Thermometers are used too often rather than too infrequently, and it is the normal pattern for children to sometimes have temperatures of little significance. There is a constant war going on between the goodies (us) and the baddies (nasty germs and viruses who are trying to invade us) and the temperature is probably just a sign that you are repulsing an attack. If you interfere in one of these minor conflicts you could in fact be helping the enemy rather than assisting the patient.

Recording a fever can be a great help in the situation where a virus infection is on the retreat and you want to know when the All Clear can be sounded; for example, in a condition like glandular fever, where you run an undulating (up and down) temperature. As it burns itself out, the temperature rises become lower, with greater distances between them and, finally, the absence of a raised temperature for a few days is an indication that the battle is over.

This sort of temperature recording should only be done on the advice and under the supervision of a doctor.

*Fever facts*

*When is a temperature a fever?* (The following are rectal temperatures, which are 1°F. above oral temperatures):

| | | |
|---|---|---|
| Under 100°F. (37.7°C.) | – | normal |
| 100°F. (37.7°C.) to 101°F. (38.3°C.) | – | borderline fever (but may also be seen in many active children during periods of emotional upset or after exercise) |
| 101°F. (38.3°C.) to 103°F. (39.4°C.) | – | Low fever |
| 103°F. (39.4°C.) to 105°F. (40.5°C.) | – | Average, or usual children's fever |
| 105°F. (40.5°C.) to 107°F. (41.7°C.) | – | High fever |
| 107°F. (41.7°C.) or over | – | Dangerous fever |

*What does fever mean?* Fever almost always means infection. A mild infection, such as a simple cold, often results in a high fever, especially in infants, while other, more serious infections may cause very little fever. Infants and young children usually run higher fevers than older children or adults with the same infection.

High fever does not necessarily mean "bad" infection, and low fever may not mean a trivial infection. Many authorities feel that fever means the body is putting up a defence and building resistance against the infection or disease. Thus, if one must be sick, the fever is beneficial unless excessive or prolonged for many days.

*What are normal fever symptoms?*

Loss of appetite.

Tired, no pep, fussy or cranky.

Headaches, other aches and pains, nausea, increased heart rate and breathing.

Change in sleep (some children sleep more, many sleep less and are more restless).

Chills, hallucinations, delirium.

*What are the dangers of fever?* The dangers of fever are frequently exaggerated. Loss of appetite is not a danger and children should not be encouraged to eat unless they want to. They must, however, drink, because, during a fever when there is an increased loss of fluid by evaporation from the skin, this fluid must be replaced or the child can become dehydrated.

A child who has had previous convulsions associated with high fevers is more likely to have further convulsions if it is undergoing some pyrexial illness and lowering the temperature in this group of children can reduce the risk. There is no danger that a fever will cause brain damage.

*When should you call a doctor?* A child with fever and no other symptoms does not need to be seen unless fever has been present for 12-24 hours. Children can get high fever within the hour, even as high as 105°F. (40.5°C), and can have thrown it off by the next morning without antibiotics or other medicine.

The presence of a fever does mean that a child must be kept under observation until the fever has subsided, and what is more important than the temperature level is the presence of other symptoms such as abdominal pain, coughing, or neck stiffness. Also, when a fever starts after a condition has been present for some days, it is usually an indication that the time has come to seek medical advice; for example, if a child is coughing for two or three days and then starts developing fever as well, this can be an indication that the disease will require more expert treatment than you can provide.

*How do you treat a fever?* The fever itself requires little or no treatment at all. The discomforts of the elevated temperature and possible accompanying headache can be alleviated by very small doses of aspirin and fluids. It is a time for observation, and the child should wear light pyjamas and bedclothes and be kept at normal room temperature. Putting too many clothes on a child (particularly a baby) can cause a temperature rise.

Do not treat a fever for more than 48 hours or give aspirin for more than 48 hours without seeking some advice. Aspirin dosage should be the minimal, and if given to children, do not exceed the dose suggested by the manufacturers.

With very high fevers tepid sponging may add to the comfort of the patient.

Do not give cold baths.

Remember that fevers most often get higher at night and are at their lowest in the morning, so do not expect a temperature to drop during the night, look for it in the early morning.

Always, with a fever, do your head to toe check for other symptoms.

*When to put to bed and when not to put to bed*

One of the commonest treatments for illness in the past has been putting patients to bed, but present medical views indicate that, particularly with children, confinement to bed finds many dangers and few advantages. This is nothing to do with the old saying that "as more people die in bed than anywhere else, it is the most dangerous place to be"! The only treatment that bed offers is rest; and is bed always the best place to rest in?

Professor Hugh Jolly, Professor of Child Health at the University of Sheffield, writes, "Is a child confined to bed against his will likely to stay at rest? My daughter aged seven was refused permission to return home on the fourth day after an appendicectomy on the grounds that she required bed rest for proper healing of the scar. The same evening I chanced to enter the Children's Ward and she had won a competition to see who could bounce up the highest from their bed!"

Professor Illingworth (*British Medical Journal*, October 1967), commenting on infectious diseases in children (the fallacies of the four fevers), said, "It has been the practice of many doctors to confine children to bed for any wide variety of conditions, such as abdominal discomfort, headache, sore throat, slight rise in temperature, a cold or diarrhoea, without any apparent reason. If a child feels well enough to be up, even merely sitting up in a chair by the fireside, and wants to be up, even if his temperature is raised, it is very difficult to think of any reason for confining him to bed. There are possible exceptions, e.g. infectious hepatitis, the preparalytic stage of poliomyelitis and the first few days of rheumatic fever."

He goes on, "I can see no reason why it should be thought likely that a child with a sore throat would recover more quickly if he sits up in bed than if he sits up in a chair reading a book in front of the fire".

It is not so many years ago that all patients after operation were kept immobile in bed for at least the first two weeks. Nowadays even after the most major operation patients are at least sitting out of bed after forty-eight hours; this is to mobilise their legs and prevent that most common and serious post-operative complication of blood clotting in the deep veins of the legs, with the risk that part of the clot will detach and rise to the lungs (pulmonary embolism).

If a child feels ill enough to stay in bed he should be allowed to do so. But if you instruct a mother to keep a child with measles in bed for seven days he probably won't want to get up for the first three, but for the last four she may have to use nearly all her and his energy holding him down between the sheets. If a child is confined to his bed in an isolated bedroom his supervision is more difficult, it is much more difficult for him to be amused and play his normal games, and most often bedrooms are the coldest rooms in the house. I can think of hardly any medical condition that prohibits a child from watching television. The only disease that might cause upset is measles, where sore, inflamed eyes will not give such a clear picture as usual. Whatever other advantages or disadvantages television has, it has been the greatest boon for ill or convalescing children.

The other reason for keeping children in bed is to keep them warm. The belief that a child with a fever needs to be kept warm dies hard. When children are ill they are more likely to be over-heated than the reverse, and one of the many reasons for convulsions in infants is that they are too hot.

It is important when a child is ill that he should not take excessive exercise, but if he takes no exercise or makes no movements his muscles will lose tone and his general body metabolism or well-being will run down. He is much more likely to get better quickly if he is activated and interested, providing it does not over-fatigue him. The difficulty in drawing the line about getting up is that "getting up" does not mean "going out", and there lies the danger, because if a child gets up after being maintained in a room at a usually or reasonably even temperature if he goes out he is exposed to fluctuations of temperature and humidity.

*Bed pans* I have a horror of bed pans. I accept that there are occasions when they have to be used, but these are rare. I think that most often there is much less physical effort getting on to a commode at the side of the bed or being wheeled to the toilet in a pushchair than the frantic balancing struggle of sitting on a cold metal sledge in a most unusual posture. This doesn't mean, of course, a trundle in the rain to the lavatory at the bottom of the garden.

The sick-room in the modern home today is not an isolated barren bedroom at the top of the house. It has become the bed-settee in the sitting-room where the child, or adult, can be supervised, and can take part in what is going on. They are part of the family, they can see what the others are eating and whether they want to join in. They are less likely to be bored there than anywhere else.

What is important is that if you send for a doctor to examine your children, you should pay him the courtesy of having your child in bed so that the doctor can have a proper look at him.

There are many reasons why confinement to bed may be harmful. It bores children, they sleep less well and there are adverse psychological and pathological consequences. In illness in children, rather than look for a reason why they should stay in bed, be looking for a reason for saying, "Why on earth shouldn't they get up?"

### *When not to send your child to school, or when to send your child to school*

Often the decision as to when we send our children to school is taken for us. Infectious diseases have laid down instructions, and reference to the instructions below will give clear decisions.

| *Disease* | *Incubation (days)* | *Isolation* |
|---|---|---|
| Chicken pox | 14 - 21 | None; exclusion from school for 1 week after eruption first appears and avoid contact with susceptibles. |
| Diphtheria | 2 - 5 | Until 2 cultures from throat and 2 from nose fail to show diphtheria bacilli. |
| Dysentry (Shigella) | 1 - 7 | During acute illness. |
| Encephalitis (Arbo) | 5 - 15 | None. |
| Erysipelas | 1 - 3 | Until clinical recovery or not less than 7 days from onset. |
| Measles | 10 - 14 | From diagnosis until 7 days after appearance of rash. Schools should not be closed nor classes discontinued. |
| Mumps | 12 - 26 | 9 days from onset of swelling; less if swelling has subsided. |
| Poliomyelitis | 3 - 21 | Not more than 7 days in hospital management of patient. |
| Rubella (German measles) | 14 - 21 | None; except where contacts include a woman in early pregnancy. |
| Scarlet fever | 1 - 3 | Until clinical recovery or not less than 7 days from onset. |
| Whooping cough | 7 - 21 | Exclusion from school and public places for 3 weeks. |

Here definite instructions are given, telling quite clearly when a child can be returned to school. It must of course be tempered with the child's state of health irrespective of the number of days past its isolation period. If it is not well and is not taking proper nourishment then of course it is not fit to return. It is a question of common sense related to the written rules.

Children react to the same simple infection in a wide variety of ways.

Other conditions where the indications for keeping children at home are fairly clear are:

1. *Impetigo,* where it is terribly important that the skin should be completely clear when your child returns to school, and that they should not use communal towels.

2. *Ringworm and other fungus diseases*, where it may be possible for a child to attend school providing that the infected area is covered but, again, emphasis must be made on the use of communal towels, borrowed clothes, etc.

3. *Conjunctivitis (red eye).* There is some evidence that there is community spread here and I tend to keep children at home until they have been on treatment for 48 hours, usually an antibiotic eye ointment. I then allow them to return if the eye is improving even though it is still a little inflamed, on the condition that the full course of treatment is carried out.

4. *Athlete's foot and verucas* are not reasons to exclude children from school but reasons for taking special precautions in changing-rooms, borrowing shoes, etc., and in the swimming pool.

5. *Coughs and colds.* A more difficult group to make a decision about are children with coughs and colds. If your child has suffered a cold and cough, then it stands a better chance of getting rid of this quickly if it has two or three days in a constant temperature, i.e. at home; and, of course, as your child is infectious, keeping him away from his classmates reduces the chance of their catching some infection.

Other evidence and facts that you would collect in making your decision would be temperature, persistence of cough, the appetite, colour, etc. In the most severe cases of chest infection medical help, and probably antibiotics, will be required, in which case your doctor would advise on the right time to return to school.

These decisions are relatively easy, particularly where your child is keen on going to school.

*Abdominal pain syndrome* Great difficulties arise in the situation where you have symptoms such as abdominal pain and where there is some doubt as to whether this is being used as a reason for not going to school rather than the pain actually being the worry. There is no simple way of sorting out this problem and very often, in the process of sorting out, a visit to your general practitioner is required. Often my help is enough to resolve the situation, but according to what I find, or don't find, not infrequently I have to pass unresolved cases to the child specialist, really passing the buck and leaving it to him to say if there is in fact anything organically wrong with the child or are the symptoms a manifestation of his desire not to attend school or the basis of some other worry. The decision is never clear cut, and there may be some abdominal pain present that the additional worry or desire not to go to school blows up out of proportion.

I call this the 'Unsure Syndrome', and if you are in a situation where you think the unsure syndrome applies to your child there is evidence you should try to collect which will help you or your general practitioner to make a decision. Most often we are not trying to prove that the child has appendicitis or renal colic, etc., we are trying to prove he has not.

Facts to collect:

1. The nature and position of the pain.
2. The nature of its onset.
3. The frequency of the pain.
4. If it is related to food, if it is related to the undertaking of unpleasant tasks such as going to school?
5. The reaction after a decision has been made that there is going to be no school today. Does the pain then disappear and the child tuck in to a hearty meal?

A lot of information can be obtained and it is important because often the child that cries wolf puts himself in danger of one day presenting a pain that is significant and nobody will take any notice of it.

If in your observations you note that your child is off its food generally, that there has been some upset of the bowels or water works, and that there are fluctuations in temperature, then this is much more likely to be an organic pain that requires medical attention. What you cannot do is ignore an abdominal pain in children even if you are pretty sure it is being used as blackmail. I have had cases where both parents, myself and the paediatrician have found no reason for a child's abdominal pain and have been unable to find a cause for it, though all of us are convinced that the child has pain. What we can do is exclude dangerous organic illnesses such as appendicitis, renal stones, etc. Once having excluded these conditions, providing the child is kept under reasonable observation we know that it is unlikely to come to any great harm; but children do have glands in their stomach, as they do in their neck or under their arms, and there is no real way of detecting them other than by operation, and we do have to try to decide that the abdominal pain is more likely to be glands than an appendix.

*Headaches* Coupled with the mysteries of abdominal pain are those of headaches in children. If they are associated with septic throats, ear infections, and sinus trouble, then the decision is usually fairly easy and straightforward, and a child should be checked for any of these three conditions as headache is often the presenting feature of a sore throat, the throat symptoms not developing until later.

If there is obvious infection, the decision is clear. Having eliminated infection two further causes are inadequate eyesight (I always check children who complain of headaches for any visual troubles) and migraine, which is very common in children.

In both these cases the parents would have to seek medical advice before making their own diagnosis.

Children seem to be split up between those who would go to school if they were dying, and those who would rather die than go to school. The second group must be carefully scrutinised and no doctor minds giving his opinion regarding abdominal pain and headaches. Before presenting your child, to help the doctor, collect as much information as you can, as outlined earlier, and always take an early morning specimen of urine when you go for your consultation.

*The benefit of the doubt* If your child complains of headache or abdominal pain he must always be given the benefit of the doubt. Only when you are completely satisfied, backed by the opinion of your doctor, should you come to the conclusion that the pain is not an organic pain but an excuse not to go to school, and if it is an excuse not to go to school, then look in as far as possible to the whole school situation; most schoolmasters are sympathetic about this problem and it is lack of consultation that prevents these problems being resolved.

*When not to call the doctor, and when to call the doctor*

There is no need to call your doctor out at three o'clock in the morning to get him to decide whether your baby is still likely to have a squint when he grows up, or to look at the mild eczema he has had for the last three weeks. These conditions, like most skin complaints, rashes and spots, can safely wait till the next day, when you can either take him to the surgery to be seen or, if infectious, ask your doctor's advice on the telephone. What you must look out for are the potentially serious complaints, like pneumonia, appendicitis, ear infections and severe diarrhoea.

If your baby or child looks ill and is very hot and has difficulty in breathing, don't try to make your own diagnosis—you need medical help.

The following conditions should be seen by a doctor as soon as possible.

1. The sick child who complains of abdominal pain and who is tender to pressure in the right lower abdomen is an appendicitis suspect. Temperature in the early stages of appendicitis is no guide to the actual condition.
2. A persistent earache, particularly with temperature, could be the sign of a middle ear infection. An antibiotic given early enough can soon put this right. If left unattended, it could lead to more serious infections.
3. Severe diarrhoea, particularly in small babies, is a potentially serious condition, because of the loss of fluid from such a small body.
4. Headaches accompany most infectious diseases as well

as conditions like tonsillitis or influenza. But a severe headache in a child who has no other symptoms may be of some significance.

5. Convulsions are perhaps the most frightening experience mothers can have with their babies or children. Although they are usually over before the doctor arrives, it is always wise to call him. He may be able to prevent further ones occurring, and will want to look into what has caused them.

Obviously for serious injuries such as broken bones, or head injuries that lead to unconsciousness or heavy bleeding, you must send for the doctor.

As a whole, it is impossible to lay down simple rules as to when or when not to call your doctor. The important thing is to think before doing so.

What are the signs that point to whether your baby or child is ill?

First, babies. The new baby has to do several things. He has to take in food and put on weight; empty his bowels and pass water, spend a large part of his time sleeping, and breathe regularly and at a reasonable rate. If he is doing all these four things, you can generally assume he's pretty well. If he is unwell you can expect him to be behaving oddly in at least one of these departments. On the other hand he could be behaving oddly in all four and still not be ill.

What points can you look for that will help? Have a look at the baby. Is he laughing and happy? Because if he is, he is probably well. Does he look ill? Has he been sick? Is he really sick and how much, or has he just brought up a little overflow at the end of the feed? Is he a good colour? Are his motions regular and normal? These are bound to have colour changes, but if there is a slight colour change is baby unhappy about it? Is the motion really different from usual?

If the baby is hot and perspiring, make sure that this is not due to his clothing and surroundings. If he has got six blankets and five vests on, and there is a four-bar electric fire burning in the same room, he will certainly be overheated and will probably have a rash. Try removing some of these things and see if the rash disappears.

If he is crying, how long has he actually been crying? Is it really hours? What sort of cry is it? Have you looked into the reason why he might be crying? Is he hungry? Are you giving him enough food? Has he got a pin sticking in him? Is he sitting on a hot water bottle? Is he too near the fire? Is some noise upsetting him? Is his nappy too tight? Are you giving him too rich a feed mixture? Are you feeding him and then putting him down straight away? Or have you brought up his wind? Are you trying to push him along too quickly and giving him sausage and chips before he has learnt to suck his bottle?

All this comes under "taking stock", and helps to rule out any panic element you might have in assessing whether there is something really wrong.

Once past the baby stage and on to the small child, there are many things you can cope with on your own.

All cuts, for example, look less terrible after they have been cleaned up and some direct pressure has been applied to the bleeding. Simple first-aid treatment should cope with the minor cuts. If there is any doubt about excessive bleeding or the need for stitching, then you must send for aid.

Constipation in a small child is not an emergency and dealing with it should be within most mothers' scope. A properly balanced diet and mild aperients should prevent you having to take your child to the surgery.

Nose bleeding generally has little significance. If you sit your child up and apply direct pressure to the nose, and a cold pad on the bridge of the nose, most nose bleeds will stop. If it still won't stop then plugging the nostrils with cotton-wool and applying firm pressure will stop nineteen out of twenty, but don't take the plug out too soon.

If three out of four of your children have either chicken pox or measles or mumps and your fourth child starts developing the same symptoms, there is no pressing need to call your doctor out that night. Most of the infectious diseases can wait till the next day.

Small burns, mild sunburn, ringworm, thread-worms—none of these is an emergency.

The ideal time to call your doctor if you need him is

between 8.30 a.m. and 10 a.m., so that he can fit your visit in with other visits in the vicinity. I know it is not always possible to get your call in at this time, but do try. Remember, too, that trying to catch your doctor during his lunch-time invariably gives him indigestion.

If you are desperately worried about yourself or any of your family, for whatever reason, then consult your doctor. Worry is a frightening, demanding, exhaustive and infectious thing, and until you can be reassured you will continue to worry. It is a disease of its own—so do try not to.

# 3

# *Management of constipation*

Constipation plagues many people throughout their lives and is a common disorder affecting every age group. The first steps in management are to take a healthy, balanced diet which includes fresh vegetables—important both for the bulk and their laxative qualities. What is just as important is to have an adequate fluid intake—the simple drinking of an increased amount of water is often enough to relieve constipation.

Having ensured that the diet balance and fluid intake are normal, then one should seek other causes.

### *The treatment of constipation in babies*

For babies the treatment of constipation is usually simple. An increase of sugar in their diet is usually sufficient to relieve constipation. It is particularly important that they are given plenty of water to drink if they have a tendency to constipation and to get things going, rather than to give laxatives by mouth. After all, unplugging the nozzle rather than squeezing the tube is the best way of getting your toothpaste out if it dries up at the end! Similarly, with babies, a small glycerine suppository will be sufficient generally to clear the lower end of the bowel and the diet, sugar/fruit regime, will ensure a reasonable bowel action.

### *The treatment of children and adults*

Where, in spite of a balanced diet—plenty of fruit, fluids, vegetables, etc.—constipation persists, the present popular choice of treatment is the use of bran. This can be bought in commercial breakfast preparations or from health food stores and in most cases is sufficient to give a regular comfortable bowel action and is probably the substance of choice. By trial and error the patient taking bran will find out what quantity he will require daily to keep a regular bowel action. What must not be neglected, and it is an important factor, both in the causing of constipation and in the relieving of it, is exercise. A healthy, athletic person is much less inclined to have constipation than somebody who does not take exercise. This is not just because of the better metabolism of foodstuffs but the purely physical action of the abdominal muscles and the movement of their intestinal contents.

For the few remaining patients who are still constipated in spite of a bran diet, etc., the more conventional laxatives have to be used and there is a wide variety and choice of preparations with the vegetables perhaps being the ones of choice. In all cases where severe constipation is being treated, as in babies, freeing the lower end is most important. There are a wide variety of ways this can be done:

1. A simple glycerine suppository which acts as a lubricant.
2. Various commercial suppositories that act more in the way of an enema suppository combined and usually cause a vigorous bowel action itself.
3. Bowel wash-outs (enemas), which should only be given by somebody who is trained in this procedure.

Enemas are only really called for in the situation where there is immobility of the patient, such as the ill or elderly and infirm, where the normal muscular exercise of getting about is not carried out and this aid to emptying the bowels missed.

In treating constipation of the elderly and infirm, encouraging them to go to the limit of their exercise tolerance could be most helpful in combating constipation.

Certain medical preparations and treatments can themselves give rise to constipation, especially any morphine derivative. Report to your doctor who is treating you if you note that you are becoming constipated after starting a particular treatment and he can tell you whether it is related to that treatment and may be able to make some adjustment.

4

# *Management of ear troubles*

When your child, who has always been relatively well behaved, stops coming when you call him, it does not mean that he is on the pathway to delinquency, it is most likely that he hasn't heard you.

Being aware of hearing problems in children is always difficult as often it is related to winter colds, or throat and ear infections, and the only obvious symptom might be that he demands that the television and radio are turned up even louder than usual.

Schoolchildren have routine medical examinations which include the inspection of ears and also, when required, audiometry tests to ascertain hearing levels and ability. A cold or an ear infection a week after the examination could leave a child markedly deficient in hearing. Not hearing well could make him inattentive in school, as he may never quite hear exactly what is being told him, either in directions of what to do, or simply muddling up of figures, like five and nine, as his hearing is not acute enough to differentiate clearly. Often a child whose schoolwork starts to fall off and who becomes lazy and dreamy just cannot hear well enough to be involved in what is going on. The loss of hearing ability can be slow, so the corresponding raising of voice to compensate and get through is insidious, and is not noticed.

If hearing problems are not attended to they can deteriorate and, in some cases, actually lead to deafness. Every winter thousands of children have ear infections and colds that can affect their hearing. Sometimes this is of a temporary nature, but at other times it persists, affecting the child's general response to noise, and is sufficient to interfere with his general attention and concentration.

Before antibiotics were available ear infections were a common worry, and some danger, perforated eardrums and infected mastoids often being the outcome. Happily, since the availability of antibiotics, the number of perforations and acute mastoid infections is a fraction of what it used to be, and that fraction is steadily getting smaller. What is seen, however, more frequently since the advent of antibiotics is a condition best described as "a gluey ear". When an ear infection is present it is usually accompanied by pain, often temperature and other symptoms, but if the infection is killed by antibiotics, the symptoms disappear and the child can be left with a collection of this gluey, catarrhal, material behind the eardrum. It is this collection of glue that is one of the main causes of hearing loss in children. It presents the same sort of situation as the opening of an airtight can. You cannot open many airtight cans until you have pierced a hole in the lid and, similarly, the glue won't drain away down its drainage channels until some air can get behind the drum to fill the space it was occupying.

Once a gluey ear has been diagnosed, it can be treated. One treatment is, make a small incision into the eardrum (myringotomy) and take the glue or fluid away. Associated with this, and more commonly (increasingly so for the last 10 to 15 years) has been the insertion of small plastic tubes called grommets into the eardrum. These allow sound and air to pass.

The number of children having this procedure carried out each year is increasing, the results are sudden and dramatic, and most have no further ear troubles. No treatment can be started without the condition first being diagnosed. Only inspection of the eardrum and audiometry can show actual hearing losses.

The way to prevent and be aware of ear troubles is for parents to follow some simple rules for the ears.

1. Inspect ears at washing time, remove superficial wax in the outer ear with cotton wool. Inspect ears for discharge or skin troubles in and around the ears.

2. If you suspect any trouble with the ear, have it looked at. A very common cause of temporary loss of hearing is blockage of the ear with wax. Some people produce more wax than others. It is nothing to do with any deficient standard of personal hygiene. This wax can only be removed from the ear by syringing of the ears. Syringing of the ears must be done under medical supervision and provides dramatic and immediate relief.

If your ears do require to be syringed then it is likely you are an excessive producer of wax and it is advisable to have your ears checked up and properly syringed every one to two years.

Do not try to poke wax out of ears with matchsticks, hair grips or your car keys. They can damage the ear, or cause infection and, anyway, cannot get down to the wax deep in the ear canal. Hard wax, as well as interfering with hearing, can complicate ear infections by preventing them from draining and, as a result, in time, can cause the drum to be damaged; so it is important that if ears are blocked with wax, they should be syringed clear.

3. If your child has earache, even if it gets better, have his ears inspected by your general practitioner. The fact that the symptoms have subsided does not mean that no treatment is required, and a chronic low grade condition can build up into an acute one if not treated.

I always inspect children who have had ear infections a week after they have started their course of antibiotics. It is not enough for the child just to feel better—the ear must be looked at to see that the infection is completely cleared.

4. Do not, if started on a course of antibiotics for earache, stop when the earache goes. All prescribed courses of antibiotics should be finished to the end of the course. If the course is stopped halfway through it could allow the germ that is being treated to become resistant to the antibiotic and further infections may not respond to treatment. A simple explanation of the use of antibiotics is that they can be compared to a truncheon hitting the germ on the head. Once the germ is unconscious the signs and symptoms of infection disappear and it is no longer active, but unless

the beating is continued until the germ dies, he will recover and from then on, having recovered, will have a thicker skull. The next time he has to be beaten it is a harder job to make an impression on this thickened skull and a heavier truncheon may have to be used.

This use of antibiotics applies not only to the treatment of ear infections but to all infections where antibiotics may be used. The temptation to stop the course is perhaps greater in the presence of an ear infection as there is nothing to see and, when the pain has gone, one is likely not to bother so much.

5. All discharging ears must be inspected by a doctor.

Do not put in oil drops or plug with cotton wool. They are not sterile and, because they are not sterile, they can be a cause of infection themselves.

Do not use the ear drops that are still in the house from the time when Auntie Kitty had ear troubles. They may be no use for the particular infection that is being treated; they may be out of date in their usefulness, and they could also have become contaminated and be an actual source of infection themselves. Only use ear drops that are prescribed by a doctor, under the directions of a doctor.

6. If you suspect that your child has some hearing difficulty, carry out a simple hearing test:

(*a*) Speak to him from behind when he cannot see your lips moving or what you are doing. This often gives quite a clear indication of poor hearing.

(*b*) Compare the two ears by holding a faintly ticking watch to each ear and see if it can be heard on both sides.

(*c*) See at what distance he can pick up your whisper, aiming to test both ears by whispering from different distances and either side of the head.

If, following tests, you are uncertain of your child's hearing ability, seek medical advice.

7. If you find your child is becoming withdrawn and inattentive at school, carry out simple hearing tests and if you are not satisfied that his hearing ability is perfect, seek medical advice so that he can have his ears inspected and, possibly, audiometry tests conducted.

*First aid for ears*

1. With foreign bodies such as beads or insects in the ear, do not attempt to remove them by probing with a hairpin. If they do not come out with shaking the head on one side, then they will have to be syringed out by your doctor or nurse.

2. *Bleeding from the ear* following a head injury. This is the one first-aid situation where you do not try to control the bleeding by pressure. If there is bleeding from the ear following a head injury, you must consider that the base of the skull has been fractured, and treat accordingly until proved or disproved by X-ray examination.

*Be ear conscious*

Our ears are two of our most precious possessions, so if Tommy doesn't come when you call, and your television can be heard all the way down the street, make sure you have his ears looked at.

*5*

# *Management of infection*

When disease is caused by the action of micro-organisms or germs it is said to be an infection; the word also has the connotation of people being able to pass it on from one to another. The micro-organisms concerned are mainly bacteria and viruses, although fungi and parasites come within the classification. Both bacteria and viruses are extremely small, only being visible under a microscope, but bacteria are the larger of the two and attack human tissue from outside the cells, whereas the smaller viruses are able to penetrate right into the cells and so are harder to get at and eliminate. Not all germs are harmful to humans. There are germs on our skin and in our gut with which we live quite happily under normal conditions.

Infectious disease is usually caught by breathing in germs that an infected person has breathed out. Every time breath is exhaled a fine spray of droplets of moisture is spread in the air around. The droplets carry germs and they hang suspended in the air for a considerable time. You can see evidence of this when breathing on a window pane, or in the way breath forms a fine mist in cold weather. If the breath is exhaled forcibly, as in a cough or sneeze, the germ-carrying droplets are spread even further. This is the way the winter influenza and coughs and colds are spread around crowded places, such as cinemas or buses. By coughing into a handkerchief much of the water vapour is trapped and so infection is cut down. Some diseases need actual bodily contact for infection to be passed on, and these diseases are said to be contagious. Not everybody who comes into contact with infectious diseases necessarily catches them. So whether a disease is caught after contact depends not only on the amount of exposure to infection, but also on the susceptibility of the recipient.

The first line of defence of the human body is mechanical. The intact skin and linings of the breathing and food tract form efficient barriers to infection. The outer surface of the skin consists of a horny layer of dead cells being shed constantly, which organisms have to penetrate before reaching the more susceptible living tissues underneath. The membranes in the nose and repiratory tract are lined with minute hair-like processes called "cilia" which are in constant motion. These act like a fly-paper and catch inspired organisms which are then conducted by the wave-like movements towards the exterior. The membranes are also washed by secretions of various fluids such as saliva in the mouth, tears in the eyes, and the moisture in the nose. When infection threatens these secretions increase, which is why we get a runny nose with a cold.

If the skin is broken or the organisms are sufficiently powerful to overcome the local defences and gain a foothold on the membranes themselves, the defensive cells of the blood—a particular type of white cell—are rushed to the area and the blood supply to the area itself increases, making it warm and red or, as we say, inflamed.

The white blood cells which conduct the defensive action are called phagocytes or eating cells because they are able to flow round and destroy the invading organisms.

If a blood sample is taken from a patient undergoing infection, the proportion of white cells is found to be greatly increased in response to the threat. There is also a system whereby any protein which is foreign to the human body, such as in invading organisms, is isolated and neutralised so that it has no harmful effects. The foreign protein is called an antigen which in turn induces the recipient to produce an antibody. These two combine to produce a neutral substance which does no harm and can be eliminated.

The ability to produce antibodies has to be learnt and this depends on the host having met the specific antigen before. In the course of a first time infection the antibodies take a considerable time to be produced. If the antigen has been met before the production mechanism is familiar and the right antibodies are quickly brought into production. If some time has elapsed the mechanism is not quite so familiar, and so their production is not quite so quick. This explains the phenomenon of immunity which varies from disease to disease. If a cold is caught in the winter usually there is a period of relative immunity lasting a few weeks or so, but after this time the immunity deteriorates and another cold can be caught. This is a short-lived immunity, whereas one is very unlucky to catch the common childhood illnesses of measles, chickenpox or German measles more than once; in other words the immunity conferred by an attack is usually lifelong. The ability to produce antibodies is hereditary to a certain extent. In the first year of life when babies are at their most vulnerable in many respects it seems that Nature has given them a protection transferred from the mother so that, during this period, it is unusual for the childhood illnesses to be contracted or, if they are, only very mildly. Sometimes an infection so mild that the disease goes unrecognised is enough to give lifelong immunity.

Many people go through life without developing a proper attack of mumps, despite close contact, and it must be assumed that they have had at some time a sub-clinical attack which protects them thereafter.

If a whole race of people have never met a disease before, the ability to produce adequate defences is very greatly diminished, and so a disease which is relatively benign in an area where it is common can be disastrous in a new population. When the Europeans first went to Polynesia, they took with them measles, which had not been known there previously, and it caused a very severe disease which killed many people.

Immunity can be artificially induced by inoculation and it is common practice to do this now to children. At present babies are given a dose of killed or detoxified organism for the diseases of diphtheria, tetanus, whooping cough, measles and poliomyelitis, and at a later stage girls are protected against German measles, or rubella, as an infection during pregnancy can produce a malformed baby. Smallpox is not usually included now unless the person is going abroad. T.B. is done if the child is susceptible, as it is quite possible, and was common, for children to get unrecognised attacks which they overcame, and from then on were immune. The present routine for tuberculosis is for school children, at the age of 13, to have a skin test which will tell whether they have a developed immunity to tuberculosis or not. The group that have a negative response to the test are given an injection which will enable them to develop their own immunity. There is a list of other diseases which can be protected against for foreign travel, such as cholera, typhoid and yellow fever.

Inflamation of a part of the body means that a fight is going on between the invading organism and the body's defences. If this is localised, as with a boil, pus may be formed from the dead organisms and white blood cells. If the body's defences are winning, the inflamed part is well localised to one place, but infection may spread to the lymph glands, draining the area, so a boil on the hand could cause enlarged and tender lymph glands under the armpit and on the front of the groin. Red streaks of lymphangitis may be seen in between marking the course the infection takes travelling up the lymph channels. A generalised infection will produce a generalised rise in temperature of the whole body, and a feeling of toxicity. Children's temperatures rise to fairly high levels easily, e.g. 106°F. (41°C.) and they can come down again, whereas an adult with a temperature over 100°F. (37.7°C.) feels very ill. This rise in temperature, accompanied by a rapid pulse, is evidence of all the body's metabolism speeding up in an effort to fight the infection. If the temperature rises too high it may produce convulsions, especially in children. Measures should be taken to lower it. Loose cotton clothing should be worn; nylon is not very suitable. The temperature of the room should be comfortable and, if necessary, the skin should be bathed with lukewarm water; its evaporation will help to lower the body temperature. Aspirin and paracetamol are useful drugs to help lower temperature and should be used for the purpose in addition to their ability to relieve pain.

A good maxim in medicine is "Rest all inflamed parts", and this can mean anything from immobilising a wrist with a boil on it, or not giving any food to a patient with an attack of gastroenteritis, to putting a patient with a high temperature to bed.

When a fight is going on against invading organisms, the body needs all its energy to conduct this fight and so complete rest enables the body to concentrate all its energies towards this end.

A patient with a high temperature loses body moisture constantly, not only in the obvious way by sweating, but the increased respiration rate from a feverish body gets rid of more moisture. Feverish patients notice that their urine becomes darker and stronger smelling because it is more concentrated as there is less fluid to be excreted. An effort should be made to encourage an adequate intake of fluid, as a good flow of urine helps to get rid of the increased waste products of the speeded-up metabolism. An adult needs 2-3 litres of fluid in 24 hours, but this can be increased in very high temperatures. A good guide is the volume of urine, which should be 1½-2 litres per day. A lower volume indicates an inadequate fluid intake.

Appetite is diminished in the feverish state, and as long as the high temperature does not last for longer than a week or so, which is usual in most illnesses, no great harm is done. The high metabolic rate means that a great deal of nitrogen-containing tissue is broken down, and it is found that there is a considerable weight loss, but this can be made good after the return to normal health.

A diet of glucose-containing drink usually flavoured with lemon or orange, along with light foods such as soup, eggs and jellies, should form the basis but, within reason, "a little bit of what you fancy does you good".

In the last thirty to forty years, antibiotics have changed the whole outlook of treating practical infections. Until that time the body only had its own defences to cope with diseases like pneumonia, and the true value of good nursing procedures to boost these defences was more fully appreciated. Antibiotics have so greatly improved the outlook that the importance of good nursing has been overshadowed. Nevertheless, the same principles still hold true, and rest is as important in recuperation as ever it was.

Antibiotics are substances which kill off bacteria without doing harm to the host. So far little progress has been made with drugs to combat viral infection and so these diseases still have to run their course and the body defeat them on its own. Penicillin was the first true antibiotic which killed bacteria and it and its derivatives are still the safest and most widely used of antibiotics.

There is a great variety in the response of different bacteria to different antibiotics and so, ideally, the organism involved should be isolated from an infected specimen of sputum, for example, in the case of a chest infection. Having been isolated, it is found which antibiotic the organism is sensitive to, and the condition is treated with this antibiotic. This takes time, however, normally two or three days, which may be vital at the onset of a disease, and results achieved in laboratory conditions are not always relevant in the live situation in the body. So, from past experience of similar cases, the doctor will choose to give an antibiotic which he considers suitable while waiting for laboratory results to come through.

Some people react in an adverse fashion to certain antibiotics, the best known being an acute generalised rash with much swelling and itching after being given penicillin. Such people are said to be "sensitive to penicillin" or "allergic to penicillin", and once this has been established they should not be given penicillin again as subsequent reactions are likely to be more severe—to such an extent as to be life endangering. Confusion can arise as this same phrase "sensitive to" is used in the context of the invading organism, which is said to be "sensitive to" an antibiotic when it is meant that the disease will respond to a specific antibiotic.

There is a great temptation when an infection is on the mend to think that the worst is over and that the antibiotic can be done without. The reverse is often true, in that the improvement is due to the antibiotic, and if the treatment is stopped, the infection will take hold again. Antibiotics are drugs which should be taken for a time specified by the doctor, and then stopped. If they are stopped too early, there will be organisms left over which have been exposed to the antibiotic and will have learnt in part how to be resistant to it, so if the antibiotic is given again it may be found to be not so efficacious. It is important also that the dose that the doctor prescribes be adhered to. For an antibiotic to work there must be a sufficient concentration in the blood and therefore if a doctor says "one capsule four times a day for five days", one capsule twice per day for ten days is worse than useless.

The more common minor respiratory diseases which are prevalent every winter, like colds and influenza, are mainly due to viruses, and antibiotics have little or no effect on them. However, when a virus infection strikes the general resistance may be lowered and a secondary bacterial infection may develop, giving bronchitis or something similar. Antibiotics do have a part to play here and are of especial importance in elderly or infirm people or the very young, in which case an antibiotic may be given prophylactically, that is to prevent infection before it arises. Broadly speaking, the shivering and pricking sensation experienced in the nose and throat during a cold is due initially to a viral infection. If this progresses to a profuse nasal discharge, that is with yellow or green pus-like material as opposed to just a clear watery runny nose, it is likely that there is a secondary bacterial infection.

Likewise, if the material that is coughed up is yellow, green or grey, this is likely to be bacterially infected, whereas a white frothy sputum is not so infected. The above is only meant as a guide and should not be considered true in every case.

Doctors do not give antibiotics in every case as,

(*a*) The cost would be prohibitive,

(*b*) The phenomenon of resistance of organisms to antibiotics would be increased, and

(*c*) Although the common antibiotics are relatively harmless, they do have their troubles.

The human body in good health acts as a host to a variety of organisms which live in harmony with us. For example, there are a large number of an organism called E. Coli in the gut which cause no harm in their proper place. Antibiotics kill off organisms, both good and bad, and if the organism with which we live happily is killed off, organisms which are not so harmless have a chance to grow. So, after a course of antibiotics, it is not infrequent to get an attack of diarrhoea because of an overgrowth of harmful organisms in the gut taking the place of the harmless E. Coli which have been diminished by antibiotics.

So antibiotics have to be given with discretion where their use is beneficial and should not be used for every infection as the body is quite capable of dealing with minor infection itself.

There used to be strict quarantine procedures used when the minor infections of childhood were being nursed. However, in recent years, these have largely been given up. Most children still get chickenpox and German measles, mumps to a lesser extent and, until a few years ago, ordinary measles, but a vaccine is now given routinely, so measles is very much less common.

If these diseases are contracted in childhood, they are usually not too severe, so many people like to get them over with early on and so be immune in later life. Also, a sufferer is probably at his most infectious in the few days when he is starting to feel unwell, but there are no symptoms definite enough to make the diagnosis certain, and so isolation afterwards was too late anyway.

If strict control of infection is enforced on entering the sick-room a gown should be put on and taken off before leaving. Careful washing of the hands should be carried out after each contact with the patient, especially after handling heavily infected material such as dressings and bed pans. Finger nails should be kept short and hands should be washed in a dilute solution of antiseptic. If the patient is producing copious sputum or nasal discharge, ordinary handkerchiefs are contra-indicated. It is much better to cough or spit into a receptacle which can be washed out and disinfected and to use paper tissues which can be burnt.

Dust should be kept under control in the sick-room by damp dusting as opposed to vigorous sweeping, and it should be remembered that the contents of a vacuum cleaner bag will be heavily infected.

When the illness is over, thorough cleaning should be instituted, but probably the most effective measure is opening the windows wide and giving a good airing.

6

# *Common infectious diseases*

Having an infectious disease may be one of the few opportunities the school-aged child has of watching television non-stop for two weeks. For whatever instructions have been given to the patient, after two days he will either have crept down to lie beside the set, or a harassed mother will have installed the set in the sick-room.

The great exception, of course, is measles, for with that affliction sore eyes (conjunctivitis) may cause interference and a bad picture.

For the adult this is often the time for catching up with his reading matter but, by and large, adults who have what are called the children's infectious diseases in later life are hit pretty badly with them and are usually feeling too poorly to do anything else at all.

It is not always necessary to call a doctor to see the common infectious diseases. Scarlet fever and measles are notifiable diseases, so have to be seen, but, depending on the severity of the condition, chicken-pox, mumps, etc., are relatively easy to diagnose without having to call in a doctor.

*Scarlet fever*

The characteristics are a fine rash, sore throat, headache and some fever. The incubation period is from two to five days, and the interval between onset and appearance of rash one to two days.

The patient should be isolated for seven days after the rash has disappeared.

Doctors give a course of penicillin for children with scarlet fever as the disease is related to an organism called haemolytic streptococcus which can be found in the throat of patients with scarlet fever. This is the germ that indirectly can cause rheumatic fever and nephritis, so in all cases of scarlet fever a specimen of urine should be examined seven days after the onset of the disease, and if for any reason the patient is not making an uninterrupted recovery, the doctor should be consulted.

True scarlet fever is very rarely seen nowadays. Since penicillin was discovered the nature of the disease has changed; it is of a much milder form and is usually called scarletina.

*Measles*

The characteristics are sore eyes, a coarse red rash covering the face and body, high fever and cough, and the patient is usually pretty poorly for a few days before the rash appears. The incubation period is ten to fifteen days. The interval between onset and appearance of rash is three to four days.

The patient should be isolated for a week after the rash has disappeared.

Children are now inoculated against measles in the first year of life. This does not always stop them catching measles but does markedly reduce the severity of the attacks. Seven to ten days after measles inoculation some children present with very mild symptoms of measles—cough, rash, etc.—which usually clear up in a few days.

*German measles*

This is usually a red rash that lasts twenty-four to forty-eight hours. It is most often accompanied by a swollen gland behind the ear.

Patients should be isolated for seven days from the appearance of the rash. Contacts should take great care to keep away from pregnant mothers, particularly those women who are in the first three months of pregnancy.

Happily, five out of six women of child-bearing age are resistant to, and have immunity from, German measles. If they are in contact with a definite German measles case their level of immunity can be checked by going to a doctor for a blood test.

German measles caught by a pregnant mother in the first twelve weeks of pregnancy is usually an indication for termination of pregnancy as there is a high risk that there will be abnormality to the baby. It is now a general procedure to inject girls at about the age of thirteen with German measles vaccine, thus eliminating the risk of infection during early pregnancy.

### *Whooping cough*

Symptoms are a cough with the characteristic whoop, sometimes followed by sickness. Since immunisation, it may be less easy to diagnose, because immunisation may not prevent a child from getting the disease, but cuts down the severity of it.

Patients should be isolated for twenty-eight days from the beginning of the cough, and children under seven who live in the same house should be kept away from children who have not had whooping cough for three weeks after the house is free from infection.

Prolonged winter coughs, particularly when the coughing is mainly at night, when the cough is very little relieved by cough medicines and even a course of antibiotics, both in children and adults usually means this is a form of whooping cough. Often most relief is obtained with old-fashioned remedies such as steam inhalation. It can be depressing and worrying if coughs do persist, and a chest X-ray may be necessary to eliminate other causes.

### *Mumps*

Symptoms are swellings at the angle of the jaws and difficulty in opening mouth or chewing. The incubation period is twelve to twenty-eight days.

Children should be isolated for seven days after the swellings have disappeared.

Mumps in children is usually not a very incapacitating condition, but in adults can present as a severe illness with high temperatures. As well as the swellings in the region of the angle of the jaw (Parotid glands), the breasts and ovaries can be affected in women and the testicles in men, and if adequate care is not taken, may lead to sterility.

Other organs that can be affected are the pancreas gland and the brain can temporarily be inflamed (mumps encephalitis) with associated severe headache and vomiting.

It is important for the adult who has mumps to take it seriously and not be too active in the early stages of the disease as over-activity does seem to make the complications more likely and often the complications follow in a sequence, the jaw and facial swellings being followed a week later by breast or testicle complications, to be followed a week later by abdominal pain (infection of the pancreas) and headache and vomiting (mumps encephalitis).

Patients all make a good recovery from these rather frightening sounding complications. There is no specific treatment against the disease and bed rest, fluids and mild analgesics such as aspirin or paracetomal can be used.

*Chicken-pox*

This usually starts with a fever and crops of blistery spots on the face and trunk. The incubation period is eleven to twenty-one days, with about a two-day interval between the onset and appearance of rash.

Isolation should be for one week.

Children, although often very spotty, are not greatly troubled by chicken-pox. If there are a great number of spots which are scratched and they become infected, then the child requires antibiotics, both by ointment and by tablet, to get on top of the secondary infection.

Adults can be severely ill with chicken-pox. The spots can cause scarring and, again, if the rash is an extremely heavy one, antibiotics are usually given to prevent them becoming infected.

The serious disease which can look like chicken-pox is smallpox, which is to all intents and purposes unknown in this country, but in countries where it is endemic the difference in the diagnosis between these two conditions in adults is not always easy. The main characteristic difference of onset is that the main chicken-pox rash is usually on the trunk and the body with few on the limbs, whereas with smallpox the main rash commences on the limbs and the body rash appears later.

*Infectious hepatitis*

Infectious hepatitis is characterised by lack of appetite, nausea, low-grade fever and the development of jaundice, i.e. yellow colouration of the eyes and skin, with dark urine and pale-coloured stools. It is of low infectivity, but infection can be transmitted most easily from stools, and in the nursing of an infectious hepatitis case at home great care must be taken in cleaning the toilet, keeping to separate towels, and in hand washing, etc.

Prior to the onset of the jaundice there is usually a period of malaise and a general feeling of being unwell. Smokers, as the first sign, often lose the desire to smoke. It is important that this condition be investigated by a doctor.

There are many conditions that can cause jaundice—gall bladder disease, certain growths, reaction to drugs, etc. It will require blood tests to confirm that infectious hepatitis is present, and possibly X-rays to make certain it is not gall bladder disease.

If there are other cases of infectious hepatitis in the neighbourhood, and there is evidence of direct contacts, then jaundice in these conditions makes the diagnosis most likely to be infectious hepatitis.

There is no specific treatment against the condition. Rest is an extremely important factor. Too much activity during the acute phase of the disease is likely to cause an exacerbation of symptoms.

Until recently a fat-free diet was the standard treatment for patients with infectious hepatitis. The present view is that, apart from the initial stage when the patient has an abhorrence of fat anyway, what the patient fancies as a rule is all right for him to take (a little of what you fancy does you good). Lean meat, vegetables, fruit, etc., can be eaten freely. Alcohol is completely debarred and must not be taken again for at least a year after the condition has resolved.

It is difficult to tell a patient how long he is going to be incapacitated with infectious hepatitis. It is very closely associated to the severity of the disease. The shortest minimum period is probably three weeks and, in the more severe cases, can last for several months.

### *Poliomyelitis*

Poliomyelitis, happily, since the advent of efficient polio vaccine, has become increasingly rare. It does crop up, however, from time to time, on the Continent, and it is wise if you are going to visit an area where it has been reported to have a booster dose of vaccine.

It is characterised by headache, fever, stiff neck, sometimes vomiting, and photophobia, i.e. aversion to light.

It can also present as weakness in a limb from a patient who is feeling off colour.

Immediate medical advice should be sought whenever these symptoms appear as these symptoms not only are present in poliomyelitis but in meningitis where the same areas of brain tissue are inflamed.

### *Infective gastroenteritis*

There are several organisms that can cause gastroenteritis. It is characterised by vomiting, acute diarrhoea, and headache often associated with fever. Diarrhoea occurs commonly with stomach upsets and the doctor usually sees acute gastroenteritis as a diarrhoea that has not settled. It is most important to keep up the fluid balance. This is most critical in small babies who can become dehydrated very quickly, and gastroenteritis in small babies should be treated immediately and vigorously.

The causitive organism can be isolated from stool specimens and the appropriate treatment given. Outbreaks of gastroenteritis and dysentry can occur in closed communities such as boarding schools, workers' hostels, etc. During outbreaks, as well as receiving medical attention, scrupulous care must be taken with both private and public hygiene, i.e. washing of hands, crockery, and the disinfection of toilets and disposal of excreta, stools, urine, etc.

*Glandular fever*

Glandular fever is a condition characterised by enlargement of glands mainly in the neck, but possibly present in other places like the groin and axillae and a change in the blood count. The causative agent is as yet unknown, but is most likely to be a virus.

It affects children more often than adults, and small epidemics occur from time to time in schools.

The prevalence of the disease varies from year to year.

In children it usually presents as enlarged neck glands and a sore throat with white patches on the tonsils, the white patches probably being a secondary infection that has crept in while the body's main defences have been dealing with the glandular fever infection. It is only the non-recovery after a course of antibiotics that may make you suspect that it is something more than just tonsillitis.

*Fever* The presence of glands plus an increase of white blood cells gives a strong indication that glandular fever is present. The disease can definitely be diagnosed by a specific blood test called the "Paul Bunnel". Dilutions of blood serum from the infected patient have a specific action on a suspension of sheep's blood cells.

The test is not always positive until the disease has been established for some time, and it may take more than one test to get a positive reaction.

Other indications that swollen glands and temperature might be glandular fever are a rash on the soft palate at the back of the mouth, and in adults, after one week, a diffuse rash similar to that of German measles.

The condition may last a varying time, sometimes as little as a week, more commonly two to three weeks, sometimes for months.

Occasionally the condition is severe, enlarged glands in the chest can cause vomiting and breathlessness. There may be enlarged glands all over the body and an enlarged spleen.

It can cause jaundice from a hepatitis and very occasionally a cerebral upset with encephalitis. These complications are very rare and the disease as a rule gives no cause for worry.

It has a characteristic fever with a rise and fall of temperature, which may be from 100° to 103°F. Only a temperature chart gives a true picture of this undulating fever, and single temperatures, either because they are very high or because they are very low, or normal, can give misleading results. But the absence of a raised temperature over three days with an increase in general well-being and reduction in the size of the glands, is a good indication that the infection is over.

*Treatment* There is no specific treatment for the condition, but the good news is that it gets better on its own. The conditions can only be treated symptomatically. Where there is a throat infection a course of antibiotics does help, as if it has no effect on the actual disease itself, it is a protection against secondary infection.

I believe the course of the disease is influenced by rest and too much activity during the infective temperature phase is likely to prolong it.

Warm applications to glands and plenty of fluids give some comfort, plus simple analgesics like soluble aspirin for the aches that accompany the high temperature.

*Infectivity* The disease has a low infectivity and there is no need to take stringent isolation precautions, although infected cases should be kept clear of people in the home who are medically bad risks, that is to say, the young or elderly with heart or chest disease.

Cases are sometimes nursed in mixed medical wards and it does appear to pick out the odd individual, although occasionally in schools there are small epidemics.

If you or your child get glandular fever, there is no need to worry. It is going to get better even without treatment, but don't let your children start running about before their temperature is well and truly settled and their glands going down, or this could prolong the time of activity phase of the disease.

Make sure the condition is definitely diagnosed, do not try to make home diagnoses, as there are other conditions which you would not be able to differentiate from without medical help.

Glandular fever is a condition that rarely causes worry and is an excellent one for catching up with any television viewing that you might have missed!

7

# *Management of foot troubles*

Summer holidays and sunshine bring us out in the open and parts of our body which have remained covered and unseen during the winter emerge to see the light of day.

One of the parts to see the least fresh air is probably our feet, but with swimming, bathing and running across the sand, they have to come out of their winter quarters and face the rigours and dangers of the outside world.

Until we have something wrong with our feet we do not appreciate how much we depend on them and take them for granted. One blister can keep us immobilised for several days, and infections of the feet even longer.

The exposure of the feet makes them liable to infective foot conditions that, although not dangerous, can be nuisances which are difficult to clear up.

There are two main conditions that may cause trouble and are contracted particularly in the summer season. One is athlete's foot, which is a fungus infection and shows as cracks and scaly skin between the toe clefts, sometimes spreading round to the soles and sides of the feet. It itches, and the cracks may break down into wide sore splits. Another, verrucae or plantar warts, are warts similar to those that appear elsewhere on the body, but as they are on the soles of the feet, you are standing on them all the time, pushing them inwards and preventing them growing outwards. They are caused by a virus.

## *Athlete's foot*

Few athletic people go through their lives without contracting this. Swimming pools and showers are the main places where infection can be picked up. One pair of infected feet can contaminate a whole pool or shower-room floor.

Circumstances that make you more likely to pick it up are the inadequate care and toilet of your own feet. The ideal circumstances for athlete's foot to survive is a nice damp unwashed area between two toes encased by socks that are rarely changed, with the whole area of infection spread from time to time by a good old scratch.

Athlete's foot is a nuisance; it is a chronic condition difficult to get rid of, and has the habit of reappearing once you've acquired it, as well as being a source of infection for others.

Your first line of defence in the summer season is adequate toilet care. This means the adequately drying of feet, particularly between the toes, every time they get wet. Frequent washing of feet, and the changing into fresh clean socks is helpful: one should aim to wear clean socks daily.

It will help, too, if you prevent the circumstances in which athlete's foot flourishes from arising. Most swimming baths have an antiseptic pool to walk through which is compulsory before you are allowed in to bathe. Make sure you never miss it. Whenever possible after you have been in the pool, wash your feet under a tap, then dry them thoroughly and put on dry footwear.

There is nothing athlete's foot likes better than a wet sandal after a bathe, and if you allow your sandals to get with you under the communal shower, then you are establishing almost a permanent source of further infection. Don't lend or borrow shoes, and be extremely careful about the purchase of second-hand footwear.

Also make sure, particularly in foot hygiene, that you stick to your own towel—don't lend or borrow, as this is another very common source of cross infection.

If in spite of all your care you do contract athlete's foot, although there are many proprietary preparations for the treatment of this condition, I think the most effective is Whitfield's ointment. The feet should be washed each night, thoroughly dried and any flaky skin removed, then some ointment gently rubbed into the infected area.

A foot powder during the day will help to keep the foot dry. Cotton socks should be worn and changed daily. Powder your socks, shoes and slippers as well. Once you have started treating your feet, continue your treatment, putting ointment on each night for a month whether there is anything to see or not, otherwise the condition will break out again.

If too much ointment is applied too vigorously this can burn the damaged skin, so care should be taken to put on small quantities, and rub it in gently. Wash and dry the feet before further applications of ointment.

If the condition gets out of hand, or there is widespread involvement of the foot, then you should visit your doctor for more specialised treatment.

Most of us at some time have athlete's foot and it is the care and attention we give our feet, plus the safety precautions we take when bathing, etc., that determines how long we allow ourselves to suffer with it.

*Verrucae*

These are picked up in almost the same circumstances as athlete's foot. Fortunately it is not quite as infective, although it is more difficult to get rid of, and requires drastic treatment.

They show as painful hard lumps on the soles of the feet. Like warts anywhere, plantar warts will sometimes disappear of their own accord, and you can attribute this to being charmed away, an eclipse of the moon or to anything you like, but just be grateful that they have gone. For those that do not disappear you must take medical advice, or go to a chiropodist, who will treat the warts with carbon dioxide and liquid nitrogen, or cut them out. You should not attempt to do this yourself.

Now cutting a verruca out of the sole of the foot leaves a hole, and the bigger the verruca, of course, the bigger the hole and you have to suffer the healing of this hole in your foot. The earlier you go for treatment, the smaller a hole you will have in your foot to heal after treatment.

If you have one, be careful that you do not give it to other members of the household. Stick to your own towel, don't share, don't walk barefooted on the bathroom floor, and have your own standing mat on the floor, rather than sharing the communal one. Most of us at some time will have athlete's foot and verrucae, there is nothing terrible or disgraceful about them, they are just a darned nuisance.

By taking elementary precautions we can make sure that we don't pass on infective foot conditions to other people.

8

# Pregnancy and childbirth

The vast majority of confinements in this country take place in hospital or nursing homes attended by general practitioners. Home confinements have, until recently, been declining in number. But, as with all other branches of medicine, there are changes in fads and fashions, and the present views are that home confinements will be on the increase.

In European countries, Holland in particular, most confinements do take place at home, and their safety figures compare with those of any other country.

The greatest change that has taken place in the management of midwifery in Great Britain in the last few years has been the rapid discharge from hospital after delivery. Not so very long ago, by tradition, one was kept in hospital for ten to fourteen days after confinement: nowadays, in the uncomplicated case, it is very rare to stay in over a week. At least as many are discharged after 48 hours to the care of the general practitioner and midwife, and in many areas now midwives are taking their cases in to general practitioner units, delivering their own patients themselves and returning home with the mother just a few hours after delivery.

### *Where to have your baby*

The most important factor in deciding is where you want to have it. If you can be delivered in the place of your choice, by the person of your choice, you are much more likely to be relaxed, and you will then have a much better chance of an easy labour than you would if you were unhappy about your surroundings, and tense and strung up.

Babies can be born anywhere, and there are records of births in taxis, aeroplanes, trains, and pretty well anywhere where anything else can happen. Generally there are three choices:

1. A specialised hospital obstetric unit with operating theatre facilities and a large comprehensive midwifery-trained staff.
2. A general practitioner maternity unit or nursing home, where there is a resident maternity staff with probably anaesthetic facilities, and equipment for doing minor surgery, but not as a rule true operating facilities.
3. The home confinement, where you are attended by the district midwife and your own doctor.

If you live in an area where there are a reasonable number of maternity beds available, and you are expecting a first, fourth or subsequent baby, then it is desirable that you have a hospital confinement. There are only a few areas now where hospital beds are not available for first confinements and confinements for the fourth child onwards.

Difficulties that might arise during labour are anticipated during your ante-natal examinations. From these examinations, which increase in frequency as the pregnancy goes on, the doctor and midwife will get the information which helps them to decide how you will get on in labour. Unless from their examinations they find some particular reason why you should go to one of the three choices other than your own, the choice of where you have your baby rests with you.

*Unmarried mothers*

There are special maternity homes for unmarried mothers, and information about these can be obtained through your doctor and the local welfare services. If booked for one of these homes, it is usual for the expectant mother to be admitted six weeks before the confinement is due, and to remain in the home for six weeks after baby is delivered.

Pregnancy is caused by the fertilisation of the female ovum by the male spermatoza. It can take place at any period of the menstrual cycle, but is most likely when insemination takes place 14 days before the next menstruation is due.

Conception can occur without penetration if spermatoza are ejaculated into the vaginal orifice.

Ovulation usually takes place between the 11th and 16th days of the menstrual cycle. Ovulation time can be determined in the individual by taking daily temperatures through the cycle, a temperature rise of one degree in mid-cycle being the likely day of ovulation.

### *Signs and symptoms of pregnancy*

Any woman of child-bearing age who starts missing her periods must be considered pregnant until proved otherwise. The signs of pregnancy that are likely to appear after having missed the first period are:

1. Swelling and tenderness of the breasts, darkening of the nipples.
2. Morning nausea and vomiting (not usual until after the first month).
3. Hyper-acute sense of smell, and desire for strange foods like sardines with peach jam.
4. An aversion to everyday food and drink, and to habits like smoking.

### *Confirmation of pregnancy*

Forty-two days after the last period it is possible to carry out a pregnancy test on women who have missed a period. Pregnancy tests before this date are unreliable. It is difficult to ascertain whether the womb is enlarging by internal examination before the 8th to 12 week.

### *When to go to the doctor*

No pregnancy can be considered a going pregnancy unless two periods have been missed. One fifth of all first pregnancies miscarry between the first and 12th weeks, and this in no way indicates that the mother is going to have trouble in future pregnancies.

Unless there is some medical, social or economic factor, there is little point in presenting yourself to your doctor unless you have missed two periods. Do not start buying prams, cots or other items until the pregnancy is 16 weeks established.

Once pregnancy has been confirmed you will need to attend your doctor, midwife or ante-natal clinic at least once a month from confirmation of pregnancy until the 32nd week; fortnightly from the 32nd week to the 36th week; then weekly until delivery of the baby.

*Management of pregnancy*

Pregnancy is not an illness. You are often fitter during your pregnancy than at any other time, and some conditions, like rheumatoid arthritis, disappear whilst the pregnancy lasts. If you have a job it is best to keep working unless for some particular reason your doctor advises otherwise. Do not change your normal routine.

*Ante-natal clinics* By far the most important aspect of ante-natal care during pregnancy is attendance at ante-natal clinics. At the clinic you will be checked for blood pressure levels, weight gain, blood levels, blood group, and progressive development of the baby, its position and presentation. This will enable the doctor and nurse to assess how your confinement will go.

*Relaxation classes* Associated with ante-natal clinics are relaxation classes where the muscles that are useful in labour can be built up, and where you can become familiar with the stages and events of labour.

*Eating habits* As the uterus enlarges in the abdomen and presses up, causing pressure to the stomach, indigestion can make life uncomfortable. This is particularly so at night, and can be best avoided by having small, frequent meals as opposed to large, heavy ones. Sleep on three or four pillows so that the weight of the uterus is pressing downwards rather than upwards. Simple antacid mixtures taken after meals will also help to relieve discomfort.

It is an old wives' tale that eating a lot and putting on weight helps to ensure a large baby. All it does ensure is a large mother, and a large mother can create difficulties for herself during pregnancy and is more likely to have a higher blood pressure than somebody of a smaller poundage.

Eat a well-balanced, comprehensive diet of carbohydrates, fat, proteins, vitamins. Most pregnant mothers are routinely put on iron tablets by mouth through pregnancy. If weight gain is excessive, the foods to cut down on are carbohydrates, i.e. bread, cakes, potatoes, sweets, sugar, ice-cream, biscuits, etc.

*Sleep* Make sure you have at least eight hours' sleep at night. If you cannot sleep, and you are not getting adequate rest, take medical advice.

*Sexual intercourse* Sexual intercourse is best avoided until the end of the third month after conception, and again after the seventh month, until the post-natal examination has taken place six weeks after birth.

*Exercise* Take plenty of exercise, but do not become fatigued. Walking is one of the best and most suitable forms, golf and bathing are also excellent, but avoid bumpy sports like pillion riding or horse riding, and diving into swimming pools.

*Bowels* Aim at establishing a regular, comfortable bowel habit. This is best achieved by a good fluid intake, and plenty of roughage. Aperients should be avoided, as they irritate the gut. See your doctor if you are constipated.

*Teeth* If you have troublesome teeth, get them attended to early on. Dental care in the later stages of pregnancy may not be advisable.

*Clothing* When pregnant you should avoid wearing any constricting clothing and maternity corsets unless you have some abdominal weakness.

*Danger signs in pregnancy*

*Bleeding* Any vaginal loss before the fourth month of pregnancy must be considered a sign of a threatened abortion. Vaginal bleeding with pain usually means that the abortion is inevitable.

Bleeding from the fourth month onwards suggests that not

only is there a possibility of the pregnancy miscarrying, but also that part of the afterbirth is over the neck of the womb. Any vaginal bleeding at any stage of pregnancy is important, and medical aid should be summoned straight away. Immediate rest helps to prevent any potential condition being aggravated.

*Excessive sickness* Sometimes sickness of pregnancy is so severe that the expectant mother becomes unwell by having been deprived of essential body fluids. If this cannot be controlled with tablets and bed rest at home it is occasionally necessary to admit patients to hospital for intravenous fluids to replace the ones that are lost by vomiting.

There is no particular reason for this severe sickness of pregnancy. Some mothers are more sensitive to upset than others. Excessive sickness in one pregnancy does not indicate that there will be excessive sickness in future pregnancies.

*Toxaemia of pregnancy* By far the most important reason for attending ante-natal examinations is to detect early signs of mother's reaction against her own pregnancy. This condition is known as toxaemia of pregnancy. Before strict ante-natal care was practised in this country, the condition was often missed, and mothers were then exposed to the risk of the condition known as eclamptic fit.

The symptoms of toxaemia of pregnancy are:

1. Protein in the urine. This is why a urine specimen is required at every ante-natal clinic.
2. A rise in blood pressure, which the doctor records when he examines you in the ante-natal clinic.
3. Swelling of the feet or hands, or both. One can have some swelling of the legs without it being toxaemia of pregnancy. This is either because the baby is pressing on the veins at the top of the legs, or that varicose veins that were present before pregnancy become worse.
4. Excessive weight gain, headache and change in vision. These signs and symptoms can come quite rapidly in the middle and at the end of pregnancy.

If four days or a week after you have seen your doctor in

the ante-natal clinic you do not feel well, and any of these signs are present, do not wait until the next clinic, but get in touch with him.

*Nuisances in pregnancy*

*Varicose veins and haemorrhoids* Pressure of the baby on the pelvis gives rise to varicose veins in the legs and haemorrhoids (or piles), which are really varicose veins in the rectal passage. With varicose veins will be some accompanying leg and ankle swelling. This can all be reduced by taking adequate rest. It is advisable for expectant mothers after seven months, as well as having a good night's sleep, to have an hour in bed after lunch.

Varicose veins can be helped by the wearing of elastic stockings. These should be put on before getting out of bed in the morning, and removed before going to bed at night. Piles are kept to the minimum by a regular, smooth bowel action, and the use of suppositories.

*Cramp* This is a common occurrence at night in the later stages of pregnancy, and may be relieved by a sympathetic husband stretching your foot and rubbing your leg.

*Requirements for home confinements*

If you do decide to have your baby at home, the midwife will instruct you and help supply you with most of what you require. The ideal conditions for home confinement are:

1. Well-lit airy room, with adequate heating (preferably gas or electricity) near a supply of constant hot water.
2. Bed (preferably a single bed high from the ground with firm mattress.
3. Two hand bowls and one large bowl.
4. Large sheet of brown paper, and plenty of clean newspaper.
5. Small table.
6. One plastic mackintosh sheet.
7. Clean old boiled linen.
8. Pail.

9. Bedpan.
10. Large jug.
11. Two bath-towels.
12. Two hand-towels.
13. Two face flannels.
14. Sanitary belt.
15. Two dozen sanitary towels.
16. Vaseline petroleum jelly.
17. Bottle of disinfectant.
18. Nail brush.
19. Toilet soap.
20. Toilet roll.
21. Nightgowns and dressing-gowns.

If there is no lavatory on the same floor, a commode in the bedroom for the first few days is very helpful.

*Layette for the baby*

1. A cot or basket with three blankets.
2. Two underblankets.
3. Four sheets.
4. Mackintosh sheet.
5. Two dozen towelling nappies.
6. Two dozen muslin nappies.
7. Three soft towels.
8. A 3in. crepe bandage for binding.
9. Hotwater-bottle and cover—for warming cot, not to be applied directly to baby.
10. Three nightgowns.
11. Three soft vests.
12. Three warm matinee coats.
13. Three pairs of bootees.
14. Shawl.
15. Pail for napkins, with lid.
16. Safety pins.
17. Small chest of drawers.
18. Baby bath.
19. Baby soap and powder.
20. Potty.

*Preparation for breast feeding*

Preparation for breast feeding begins early in pregnancy with care and treatment of the nipples. They should be kept clean, and well supported, and a well-fitting brassiere should be worn.

If either nipple is inverted or retracted, this can be put right by gentle massage, and if necessary by the wearing of nipple shields under the brassiere. By pressing on the tissue round the nipple, this helps to push the nipple outwards. If care is taken from the beginning, even severely retracted nipples can be everted.

*Onset of labour*

Backache is usually the first sign of labour. This is constant in the background, with at first irregular contractions or pains beginning in the lower back and extending to the abdomen. These pains which are intermittent, infrequent and irregular to begin with, increase in frequency and strength as labour progresses. The baby's head descending into the mother's pelvis will sometimes imitate the onset of labour, with backache and discomfort and contractions, but instead of continuing the pain will die away.

Confirmative signs of labour are the classical "show", and the passing of a plug of mucus and blood associated with the pains. This shows that the neck of the womb has begun to open, and that labour has started.

For first pregnancies it is safe for mothers to wait until they have regularly timed pains before they go to their place of confinement. Any excessive bleeding at this stage is a medical emergency, and help should be sought straight away.

For other than first babies, the mother should go to her place of confinement as soon as she has any sign that labour is commencing.

Labour may also start with a spontaneous rupture of membranes, with a loss of fluid from the vagina. This is uncommon with first babies, but becomes increasingly common with subsequent pregnancies. Labour is divided into three stages.

1. The first stage lasts from the onset of labour until the full dilation of the cervix.
2. The second stage is from full dilation of the cervix to the birth of the child.
3. The third stage lasts from the birth of the child to the delivery of the placenta.

*The rhesus factor*

It is possible that some mothers, whose blood group carries the rhesus negative factor, will develop antibodies against their baby's blood, and the child will need replacement transfusion after birth. This never occurs with the first pregnancy unless the mother has previously been transfused with rhesus incompatible blood.

There are many factors which influence whether this condition arises, the important one being the blood group of the husband, but only one child in every 400 deliveries is affected by this condition. Repeated blood tests on a rhesus negative mother up to the 32nd week of pregnancy will determine definitely whether the baby is likely to have any trouble from this condition or not.

If all the tests are negative, then where the confinement takes place is not influenced by this factor. If the mother's blood does show some antibodies against her child, then it is essential that she be confined in a hospital unit where facilities for exchange transfusion of her baby are available if necessary.

*Phantom pregnancy*

One of the unkindest tricks that the mind can play on any woman is to convince her that she is pregnant when she is not; and to convince her so completely that her body starts imitating pregnancy. She loses her period and gains weight, and her stomach and breasts enlarge. This is a recognised medical condition called pseudocyesis—a phantom or false pregnancy.

The condition is not uncommon, and is known throughout the world. It has been reported among primitive peoples, and

Queen Mary, half-sister to Queen Elizabeth I, suffered from it. Even dogs have it.

The commonest cause is the unsatisfied desire for a child by a childless woman. She may lose her periods through this desire, or her periods already having stopped for some other reason, she may start to put on weight and her abdomen enlarge. Often the size of her abdomen is related fairly accurately to the size she would be if she were pregnant.

Phantom pregnancy also occurs in women who continue to menstruate, and in spite of the fact that they have monthly evidence to show that they are not pregnant, they still believe they are. It can also occur in women who have never had intercourse. It is even possible for the condition to reach the stage of simulated labour pains.

In the thin person, a phantom pregnancy is not difficult to diagnose, in the obese woman it may require an examination under anaesthetic or X-rays to confirm that pregnancy is not established.

*Post-natal examination*

Pregnancy and childbirth cannot be considered to be complete until a post-natal examination is carried out six weeks after baby has been born.

Your doctor will examine you internally—often a cervical smear is taken at this time, and the tissues round the vagina examined to see if they have adequately healed after stitching, etc.

It is at your post-natal clinic that family planning can be discussed, your blood pressure and urine tested, and any problems such as failure to lose weight can be gone into.

It cannot be stressed enough how important this final examination of the whole pregnancy and childbirth event is.

*Exercises for keeping fit in pregnancy*

*Standing*

1. Stand with heels and shoulders against the wall.
2. Put hand into the hollow of your back.
3. Push bottom down along the wall without bending your knees more than you have to.

*Walking* Now learn to walk with your tummy bulge held up and your bottom held down.

*Sitting* Next, sit on a chair in the same way as you have learned to walk and stand. Do this, and the ache across the shoulders and back will gradually vanish as the muscles are used properly to support the tummy bulge. Wear medium-sized heels while you do these exercises.

*Bending and lifting* It is not WHAT but HOW you lift that matters. The HOW is very simple:

1. Put one foot in front of the other, bending both knees.
2. Pick up an object off the floor. Practise with a match-box on the floor.

As you get back into an upright position you will feel your thigh muscles—not your tummy muscles—pulling your weight. Use the same method for lifting a shopping basket, or a chair. You will find your thigh muscles will lift you and the shopping basket.

*Resting* A good night's rest is essential, and a good night begins at 11 p.m. at the latest. You should also rest for a short period during a busy day. At home, after lunch is a good time; half-an-hour is enough. If you are working lie down when you come home, before you start cooking.

1. Lie on the floor or on a hard mattress.
2. Have two pillows under your head and shoulders and one or two thick pillows or cushions, rolled up to form a sausage, under your thighs as close to your bottom as possible.
3. When you are comfortable, close your eyes.

**Warning**: Do not jump up from your resting position quickly, it could make you feel faint. Use this method: If lying on your back, roll over on one side; the next movement is to roll from your side until you are in the hands and knees position, with your head down; from this position straighten arms, raising the head; then, with support of the right hand, raise the left knee, and from this position stand upright.

*Sleeping at night* As you get closer to the end of your pregnancy you must support your body properly for sleeping in order to have a good night's rest. If the "resting" position is comfortable and you can sleep on your back easily, all well and good; if not, try this way:

1. Lie on your side with two pillows under your head and shoulders and your underneath arm pulled through to the front so that your hand lies in front of your face.
2. Use the cushion you had behind your knees in front of your tummy bulge and put your top thigh on it with the knee bent comfortably.

9

# Management of feeding babies and small children

### *Breast feeding*

Mother's breast milk is the best available food for babies. All doctors try to persuade new mothers to breast-feed their babies.

The preparation for breast-feeding begins early in pregnancy with the care and treatment of nipples. They should be kept clean and well supported. A well-fitting brassiere should be worn.

If either nipple is inverted or retracted, this can be put right by gentle massage and, if necessary, by the wearing of nipple shields under the brassiere. By exerting continuous pressure on the areola tissue round the nipple, it can be pushed out. If care is taken from the beginning even severely retracted nipples can be everted.

If the mother has retracted nipples after the birth, it is possible to feed her baby with her own breast milk by expressing it and giving it by bottle afterwards, or with certain types of breast shields which catch milk leaking from the breast. Some of these have rubber nipples attached to the shield, and baby can suckle directly from them. The vacuum caused by the sucking is sufficient to make more breast milk flow into the shield.

*The essential requirements for breast-feeding are:*

1. Normal breast tissue and everted nipples (or one of the methods mentioned above).

2. An adequate fluid intake. A nursing mother cannot really take in too much fluid, and should aim at a minimum of two to three pints a day above her normal fluid intake.
3. The mother must feed herself adequately, otherwise the consistency of the breast milk will be maintained at her health's expense. She will lose more of her own bodily foodstuffs and reserves than she can afford, and will become tired, lethargic and run-down,
4. Adequate rest, for both baby and mother. Most mothers will find that for a time, once they are up and about and more physically active, the milk supply will be reduced. Increased fluid intake and more rest will put this right. The baby's food supply is much more important at this particular time than either spring-cleaning or pressing a husband's cricket flannels. Sometimes an adjustment in the feed times, for example changing from three- to four-hourly feeds, can give both mother and baby more rest.
5. It is important to check that the mother is not suffering from a disease such as tuberculosis.

Provided all these requirements are filled, and baby can suck satisfactorily, there should be no obstacle to breast-feeding.

After delivery, a baby is put to the breast eight-hourly. This helps to develop the sucking reflex, and at this time the baby obtains the fluid called colostrum from the breast. The milk supply is not established until the third or fourth day, when three- or four-hourly feeding should commence.

The way a baby is held at the breast during feeding needs to be worked out by each mother with the guiding care of her own midwife. The common position for breast-feeding is with mother sitting up supporting the baby's head with one arm and controlling the breast with the other hand.

Nipples should be washed and carefully dried before and after each feed. The baby should not be allowed to suck at an empty breast nor chew the nipple, as this leads to it becoming sore.

At each feed, alternate breasts should be used first, and the baby given ten to fifteen minutes on each. The first breast should be emptied before the baby is put to the second.

Each mother and each baby have different characteristics, and as the baby progresses, a suitable feeding routine will be established. This should be a mixture of feeding on demand and common sense.

If your friend's baby managed to do without a night feed at ten days old, and yours didn't, it just means that you are two different mothers with two different babies.

If you have a contented baby who is gaining weight, you know that breast-feeding is going satisfactorily. If, however, your baby is both discontented and not gaining weight, then you should consult your nurse or doctor.

Breast-feeding is generally kept up for six to nine months. This is because at six to nine months a baby should be getting an adequate supply of mixed food from other sources and with the reduction of the number of feeds, the breast milk tends to dry up.

If, after you have stopped feeding, your milk still comes in large quantities, you can help the drying-up process by reducing your fluid intake over 48 hours, at the same time binding the breast up firmly with a wide crepe bandage. If this does not solve the problem, then you will have to seek some aid from your doctor. The thing particularly to avoid in this drying-up process is the formation of breast abscesses, and tender, reddened areas in the breast are an indication of inflammation for which you should seek immediate advice.

### *Bottle feeding*

If, for one of many reasons, you decide that you either can't or won't breast-feed your child, the only alternative is to put him on the bottle.

Having decided to bottle-feed your baby, how do you go about it? You need dried or evaporated milk, bottles and teats, and a container for sterilising them in. You must observe elementary laws of hygiene. It is not sufficient to wipe the teat on your skirt between feeds. It is most important to wash the bottle and teat thoroughly after each feed, then to leave them soaking until the next feed in some antiseptic solution such as Milton.

In selecting a teat, you want one that will give a flow of milk that doesn't require too much effort from the baby, and on the other hand doesn't drown him. You will eventually find the right one by experimenting with several teats on your own baby.

Generally all artificial milk feeds are of modified cow's milk. Ordinary cow's milk in its undiluted form is not suitable for feeding new babies; the casein content is too high, and the sugar content is too low. All cow's milk must be boiled, diluted according to the age of the baby, and sweetened with a little sugar.

The various artificial milks available for babies vary very little. The important thing is once having settled on a particular brand you must stick to it. Any difficulties that arise are more likely to be due to the way the feed is made up, than to the variety you choose to give.

There is a difference of opinion on the advantages of starting feeding on half-cream milks (low fat content) or full-cream. There is no right or wrong. Most babies will tolerate full-cream milk from birth, most will thrive satisfactorily on half-cream for the first six to eight weeks of life, gradually changing over to full cream over a period of two weeks. If a baby is bringing back its full-cream feed, change it to half-cream. If at a week old the half-cream is not satisfying it, put it on to full.

The quantity of food given to a baby will depend to some extent on his demand. From about three ounces of made-up mixture at each three-hourly feed at a week old, he will build up gradually to about seven ounces at each four-hourly feed at five months. Your health visitor or clinic will advise you.

Bottle-fed babies do require extra vitamins and should be given daily cod liver oil or its equivalent. This should be given separately and not mixed with feeds. Vitamin C can be given as diluted orange juice. This can be started from about three weeks old.

All feeds should be mixed just before they are needed. It is never a good idea to warm up a feed that has been prepared in advance. Although you can safely leave hot water in a vacuum flask to mix the feed during the night, you shouldn't leave a prepared feed in a vacuum flask as bacteria will multiply in the warm milk.

*Routine of feeding* One usually starts off with three- or four-hourly feeds when a baby is first born and then works out, as with breast-feeding, a regular pattern that is satisfactory to each individual mother and child. There are no two babies or two mothers alike.

The earlier you can omit the 2 a.m. feed the better, because then you have a better chance of a full night's sleep. But the baby who can do without it at the third week is not any better than a baby who is still having it at five months. He is just a different baby, and the fact has no more relevance than he has got different coloured hair, eyes and a different shaped nose.

For the first four or five months the baby's main diet source is from the bottle. From then, bottle-feeds will be decreased as mixed feeding takes over.

### *Mixed feeding*

Mixed feeding consists of the addition of non-milk foods to the baby's feeding routine. Usually this is begun between the third and fourth month and, as a start, small quantities of cereal are given. Eating from a spoon may not appeal to babies, and they may prefer the bottle or breast they are used to. It is best to start feeds with cereal and then finish off with milk. It is no good filling up the baby with milk, and then, when he is nice and full and sleepy, expect him to take an interest in some new foodstuff that's offered to him.

The addition of solids and semi-solids should be begun at one feed in the day with, at first, little more than a taste of whichever cereal you give. No particular feeding time is better than any other to start off with mixed feeding.

It is very important not to push too hard, too soon, in giving a baby this fresh substance to his diet. He is only accustomed to milk, so the weaker and smaller the quantity of mixed foodstuffs given at first, the less the baby is going to object to the change.

Start off by giving small quantities of very fluid cereal, perhaps made up with the baby's usual milk, for just one feed a day. The cereal should become less fluid and more solid very gradually, and it can be introduced at two and then three feeds a day.

Once a baby has become accustomed to increased amounts of cereal, then the solid matter of his diet can be further extended. Fruits and vegetables are generally the next in order and there are many excellent fruit and vegetable preparations which can be bought for infants.

If you are giving either fresh vegetables or fruit to a baby, it is important that they be pureed. One of the first fruits a baby can have is banana. This is a good old tummy filler; it can be mashed to a fine consistency and given mixed up with milk and sugar. It is very important to have a really ripe banana, almost on the verge of going black, as banana is rather indigestible and, given in its hard form, could be a cause of colic.

When the baby is five or six months old, egg can be given, again in a very soft and perhaps diluted form. It is a valuable source of iron. Similarly, meat extracts, meats and meat soup can also be introduced into the diet round about the age of six months.

It is no good giving a baby anything that he needs to chew until he has got the apparatus for chewing. By the time he is about six months old his gums are generally hard enough to chew with, although he may not have any teeth.

At six months the baby should be taking, in addition to milk, a fairly comprehensive diet of cereal, egg, fruit, strained vegetables and meat extract. From then on the diet will increase progressively.

If a baby is still hungry after having the vital foodstuffs just mentioned, then his hunger can be satisfied with the addition of starches, such as potatoes and bread. Towards the end of the first year, meat in his diet can be varied with fish. Once the baby has got some teeth and can chew and suck fairly well, it will no longer be necessary to puree preparations, and mashed food can be given instead, which will give him something to have a go at.

From one year onwards, the baby should be managing a mirror image of his father's dinner; but it is extremely important that it should not be too lumpy, that the food should be in small, easily digested particles and that there are no hard lumps of meat or even potato that he can choke on.

Weaning a baby from the breast or bottle to a cup or spoon should not be done suddenly. As early as two months, some of the milk can be given in a cup or spoon in order to start him becoming familiar with the receptacle from which he will later have his more solid foods.

All babies will take mixed feeds given time and patience, but do give them time and don't rush.

## 10
# *Nursing of adults*

Adults, though they need less amusing than children, should not be left out of things too much. Television and radio help. There are several conditions that adults suffer from which necessitate long periods in bed, particularly coronary thrombosis, heart and chest conditions and infectious hepatitis.

Patients requiring long bed treatment at home need special nursing attention. Where possible the patient should be nursed in a single bed, with room either side of the bed for nursing attendants to be able to have proper access to him.

### *Toilet*

If possible, give the patient an all-over wash (a blanket bath) each day. Bathing should not take too long, or the patient will become tired, and it is best if two people can do it. The room should be warm and free from draughts. You require:

An adequate supply of hot and cold water.
Soap and flannels.
Towels.
Dusting powder.

*Procedures for blanket bathing* Set about the task of blanket bathing this way:

1. Strip bed and leave patient between two blankets, warmed if possible.
2. Remove night attire.

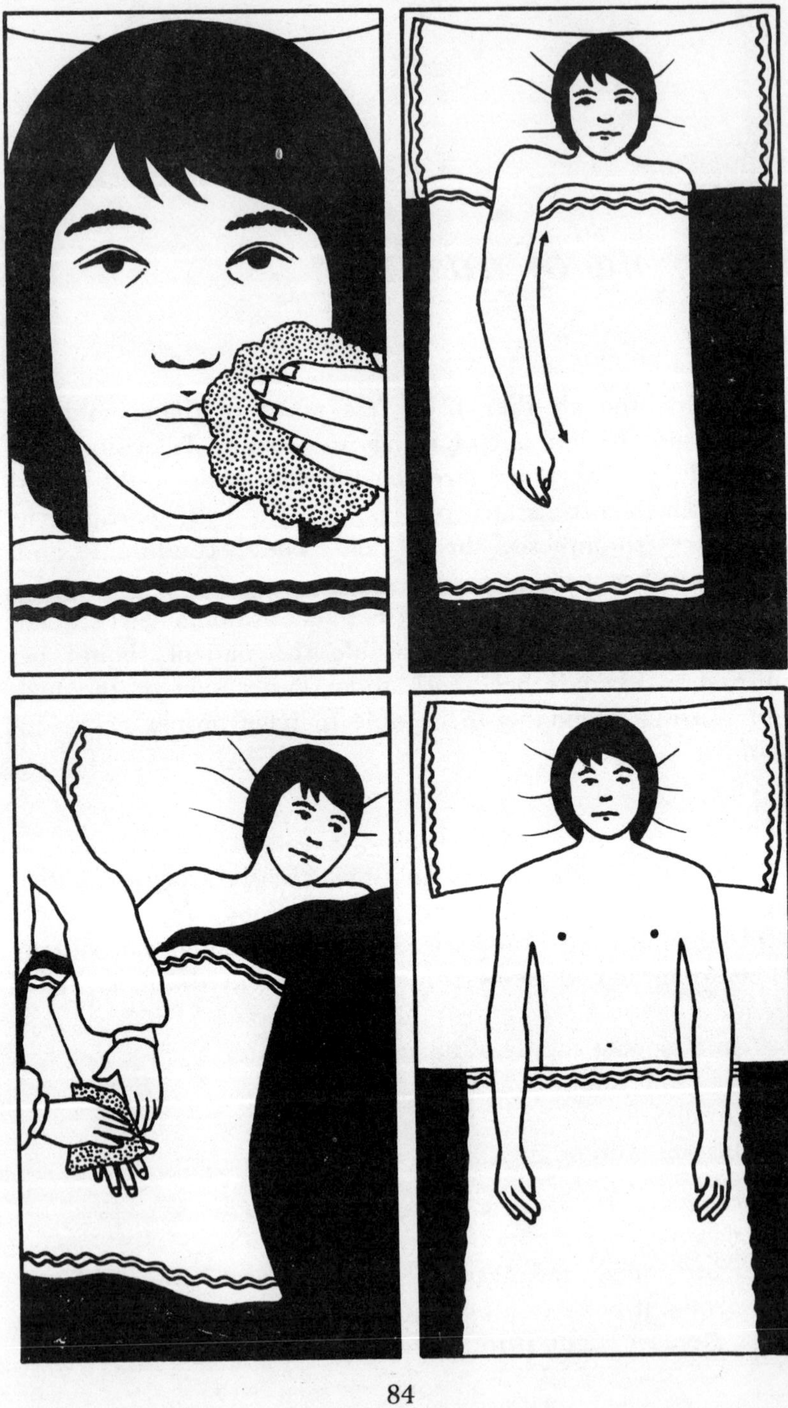

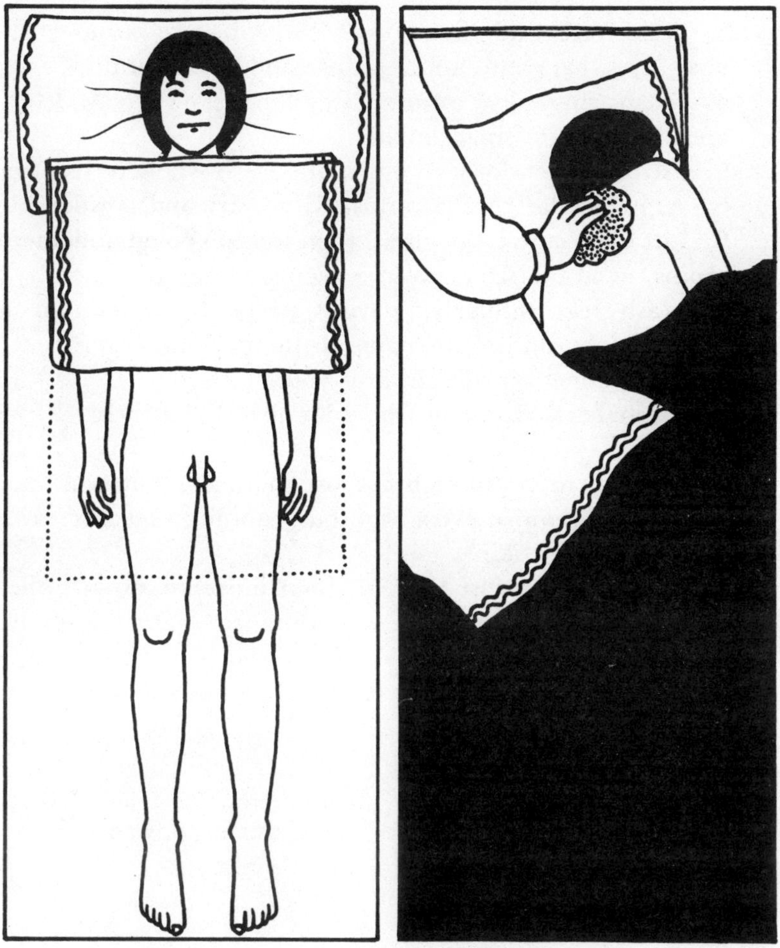

1. Procedures for blanket bathing.
1a. Attention to mouth, eyes and ears.
1b. Washing an arm.
1c. Washing a hand, care of finger nails.
1d. Washing the upper half of the trunk, with the lower covered.
1e. Upper half covered while lower half washed.
1f. The patient is rolled over and similar treatment is given to the back.

3. Wash face and neck. Take care of areas around the nose, eyes, ears and mouth. Rinse and dry carefully.
4. Wash arms one at a time, using long, slow strokes. Rinse and dry. Inspect finger-nails.
5. Turn blanket down to waist, and wash whole of front of chest, particularly under arms. Rinse, dry and powder.
6. Lift blanket to cover chest, then wash exposed abdomen, groins, genitalia. Dry, powder groins. Cover abdomen.
7. Wash legs similarly, paying particular attention in between toes, and to toe-nails. Rinse, dry and cover.
8. Roll patient on side towards you.
9. Wash back from the shoulder to the buttocks. Rinse and dry.
10. Attend to pressure areas on shoulder, buttocks and hip. These require extra vigorous rubbing. Inspect carefully for broken skin.
11. Dry the half just washed, then move round to other side and roll patient over to other side. Dry carefully. Powder.
12. Allow patient to brush teeth, clean nails and gargle if possible.
13. Put on night attire.
14. Re-make bed.
15. Give the patient a hot drink, if this is allowed in treatment.

*Bed-making*

It is best for two people to share the bed-making, being quicker and less exhausting for the patient.

1. Strip the bed by gently removing each layer of bedding,
2. Remove the sheet from beneath the blanket, leaving patient covered by blanket.
3. Loosen the under-sheet all round.
4. Remove all pillows except perhaps one.
5. Roll patient on side, giving support across shoulders and buttock. See head is supported, and patient is covered.
6. With the patient in this position, other bedmaker brushes out any crumbs, rolls the clothes close to the patient's back then attends to each piece of bed-linen in

turn, pulling it firmly, removing creases and ruckles, tucking in tightly.

7. When all is tucked in on one side, patient is rolled over to other side and the process repeated.

8. Replace pillows. Lift patient into sitting position, and fluff up pillows.

9. Replace top sheet. Remove covering blanket, then proceed to make bed normally, tucking in blankets.

*Lifting*

To lift the patient in a sitting position, two people should first adopt a correct posture of straight-back bending entirely

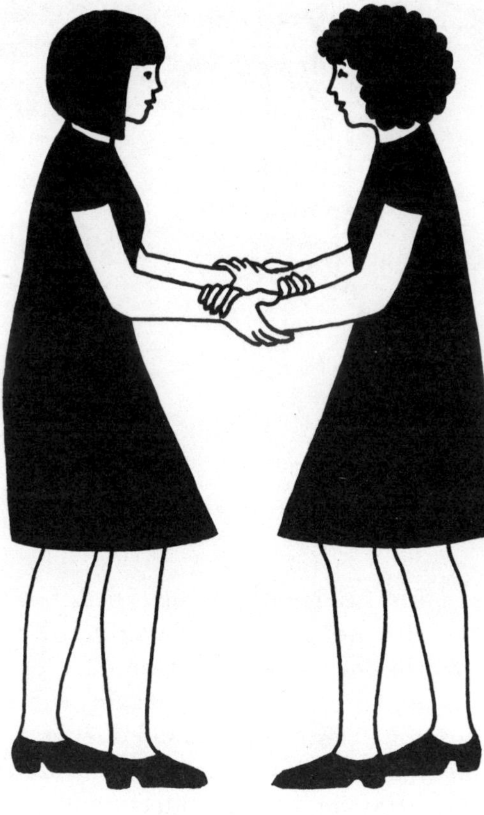

2. Hand position for lifting the patient

from hips to knees. Then they stand facing each other with feet apart. They grasp each other's wrists, with the lower arm under the thighs near the patient's buttocks, and the other arm low against the back, with the patient sitting in the well.

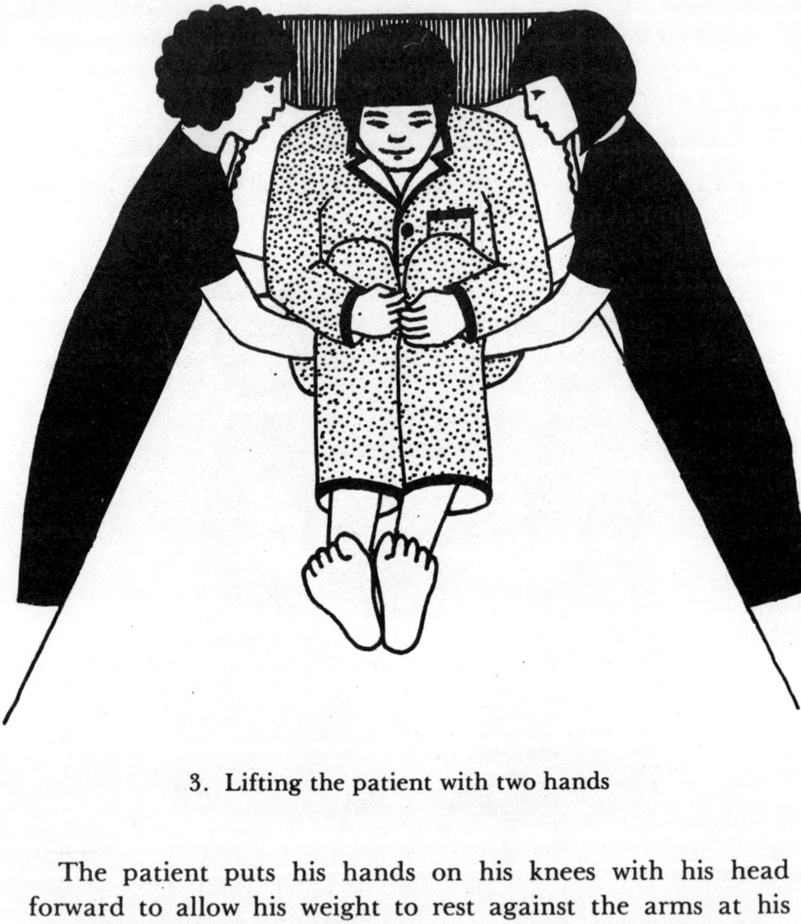

3. Lifting the patient with two hands

The patient puts his hands on his knees with his head forward to allow his weight to rest against the arms at his back. He is lifted in one movement, then back up the bed.

Alternatively, use the shoulder lift. Again with the patient in a sitting position, two people stand facing towards the head of the bed, and join wrists under the buttocks. The patient puts his arms on the shoulders of the lifters, and again he is lifted in one movement.

For the heavy and awkward patient there are many lifts and hoists that can be attached to the bed to aid his movement and management.

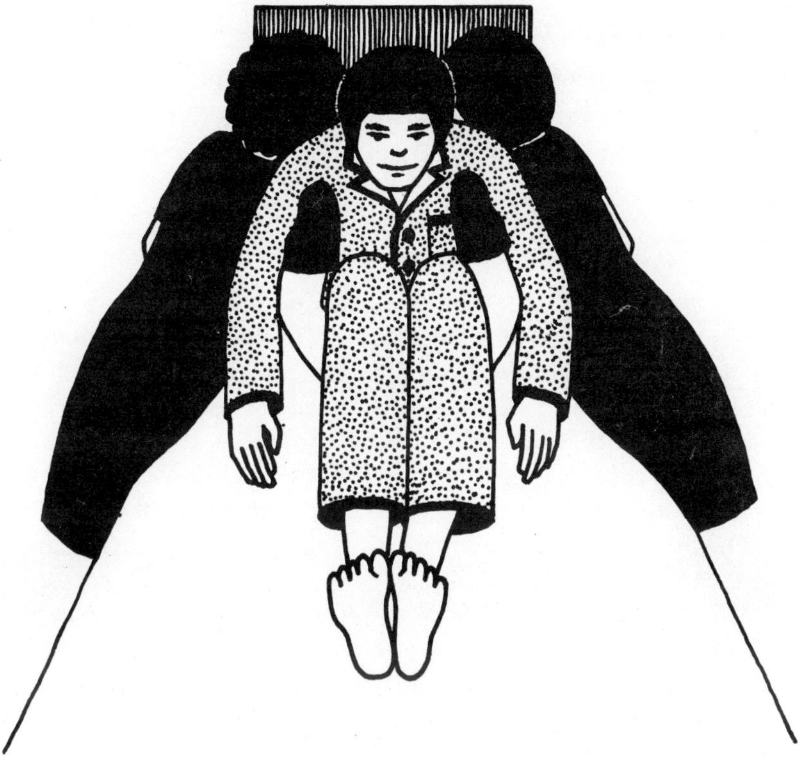

4. Lifting the patient with one arm each

*Bed-pans*

A bed-pan is not often necessary. It usually involves less physical effort to get on to a commode beside the bed, or be wheeled to a lavatory, then for the patient to have to balance in bed on a cold bed-pan.

*Bottles*

A plastic urinal bottle is essential for the male sick-room.

The breathing rate, the pulse rate and temperature are three important measurements in the nursing of sick adults. These should be kept on a chart as illustrated.

*Respiration rate (breathing rate)*

The number of breaths that a patient takes in one minute is the respiratory rate. A normal adult breathes 15 to 18 times a minute.

*Recording the pulse*

Recording the pulse is a valuable aid to diagnosis and assessment of the patient's condition. The rate and regularity of the pulse is one of the indications of the efficiency and health of the heart. To take a pulse, feel below the base of the thumb with your index finger and count the number of pulsations that you feel over a period of one minute. This will give you the heart rate and, in adults, can range from 60 to 80 beats per minute, whereas in a young baby the normal rate can be 140 per minute.

Do not take the pulse with the second finger of your hand as this has a pulse on its own and you could be recording your own pulse rate. The pulse can also be recorded from the artery at the temple, just in front of the ear, the carotid artery in the neck, and directly from the heart itself.

A rise or fall in pulse rate can be important medical evidence, to be reported. For example, in internal bleeding a rise in pulse rate would indicate the likelihood of further bleeding, and in head injuries a fall in pulse rate is an indication sometimes that there is bleeding in the brain. Exercise and excitement both put the pulse rate up. A common condition that causes anxiety is episodes of very rapid beating of the heart (paroxysmal tachycardia). This is not a sign of a heart disorder, and quite often reassurance is enough to reduce the rate, but if it persists the person should have a medical check and possible medication to maintain the pulse at a lower rate.

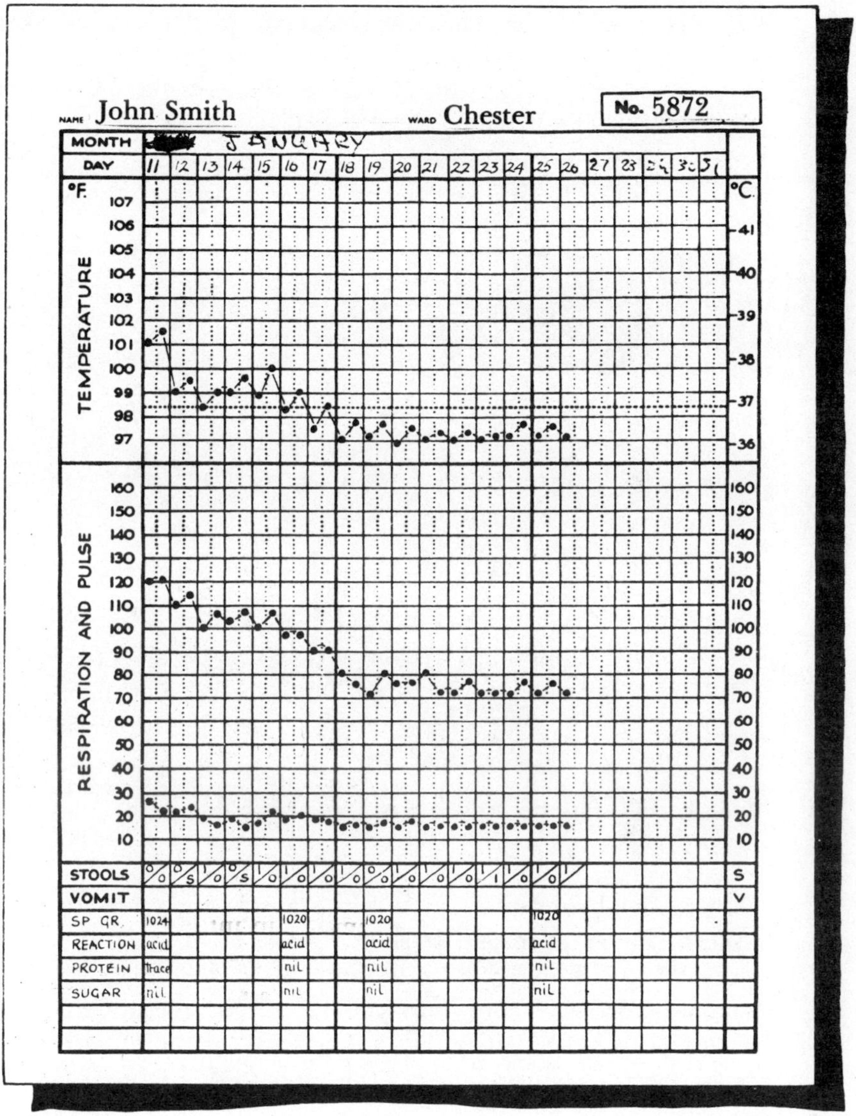


5. Temperature, pulse and respiration chart

In recording the pulse either:

1. Record pulse rates at set time intervals, or
2. Record the pulse on a simple graph so that an overall picture of what is happening can be observed.

*Taking the temperature*

A patient's temperature is one of the indications of their general state of health and its accurate recording is vital in

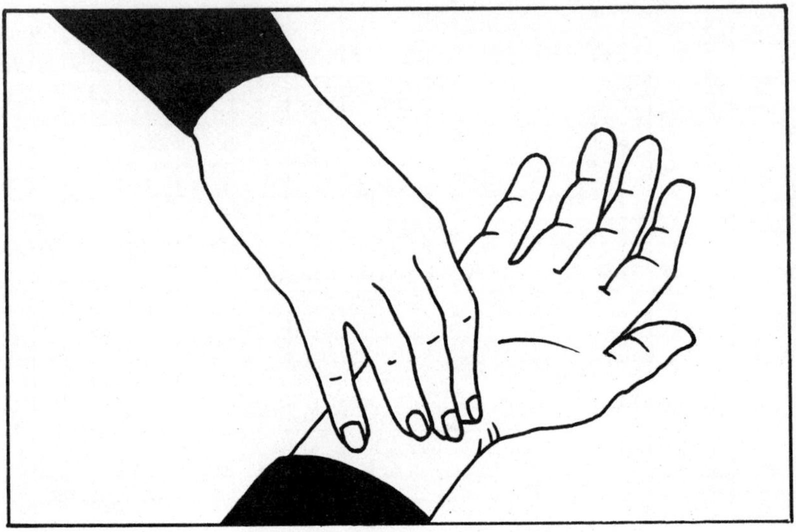

6. Feeling for the pulse below base of thumb with index finger

many medical conditions. It is important to know how to use a thermometer properly. It should be kept in an antiseptic solution, rinsed in cold water and dried before use, and shaken before it is put into the mouth or rectum of the patient so that the mercury is down in the bulb and not registering an abnormal temperature before it is used. It is too easy to have a thermometer near a radiator and record a high temperature where one is not present.

*Taking temperature by mouth* Place the thermometer under the tongue of the patients and ask them to hold it with their closed lips and not their teeth. Leave the thermometer in place for two minutes, then take out and read. The highest point to which the mercury has risen is the temperature which is recorded. At the present time the conversion from Farenheit to Centigrade on most thermometers causes some confusion. The diagram below, and table, give a simple conversion.

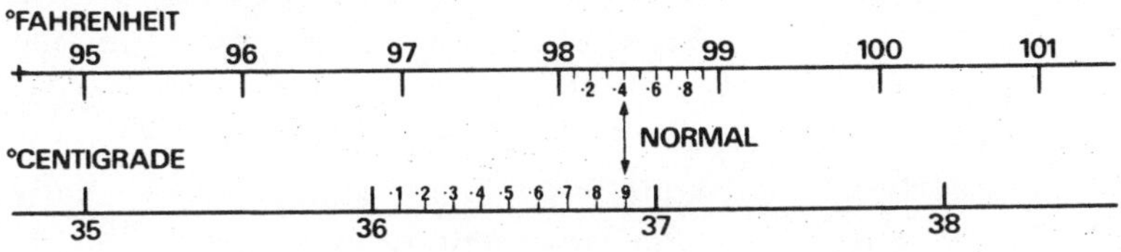


7a. Centigrade/Fahrenheit conversion scale

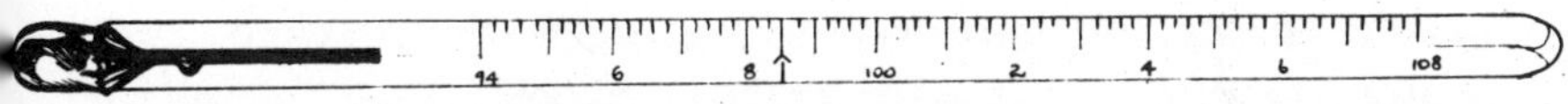

7b. A clinical thermometer

*Rectal temperatures* The thermometer should not be put into the mouth of a child who is likely to bite it, and for small children and unconscious patients a rectal temperature should be taken. Rectal thermometers are stouter than the normal thermometers used in the mouth and should be greased before being inserted into the rectum and held firmly in position. They should be read and recorded after removal, then thoroughly washed, shaken down, and replaced in antiseptic.

*Other positions* It is possible to take the temperature under the arm or in the groin. Place the thermometer into the armpit and fold the arm across the chest, or place it in the groin and cross the leg over the thermometer. When taken in either of these situations the recorded temperature will be about 1°F. below the actual body temperature, and this should be allowed for. The normal body temperature is between 97°F. and 99°F. (36° to 37°C.). A rise in temperature indicates the body's reaction to infection and is one of the aids in repelling most infections.

*Hypothermia* This is a condition that will arise when the body temperature falls below a certain minimum level. This occurs mainly in the youngest and oldest age groups. The body temperature of small babies and the elderly who get over-exposed to cold may fall to a level at which the body cannot function properly. This is an extremely dangerous condition and is frequently missed. The range of temperatures encountered in hypothermia cannot be recorded on the normal clinical thermometer and a special thermometer is required for this lower range. The condition can be recognised by the lethargic, cold, blue, semi-conscious baby or elderly person and the treatment is to warm the whole body up slowly. Do not place warm objects, such as hot-water bottles, round extremities. When possible, give hot drinks, cover the baby or adult with warm blankets and watch carefully. In the elderly hypothermia is often associated with malnutrition and the whole situation of the person found in this condition will have to be assessed and a period of hospitalisation is essential until the initial crisis is over.

Hypothermia in babies is an extremely serious condition and expert medical help will be required after the intial first aid procedures of warming the baby have been carried out.

# 11
# *Management of coronary thrombosis and the cardiac patient*

The ordinary man in the street looks on the heart with a sense of awe, he does not just consider it as an organ in the body doing an important job, but it has a slightly mystical significance as the "seat of the soul" or some such ill-defined concept, and hence anything to do with the heart is viewed rather more emotionally than, say, the liver, which is just as important but not quite so dramatic.

Nevertheless the heart's function must be understood just like any other organ and can be conveniently thought of as a pump. The bulk of it is made up of muscle, a slightly abnormal type of muscle in that it keeps contracting and relaxing quickly, day and night, without any rest. Like any other muscle it requires a blood supply to give it nourishment to provide energy for its ceaseless activity; the blood supply also takes away the waste products that are left over from this process. Where the main blood vessel—the aorta—comes out of the left half of the heart, two small blood vessels, the coronary arteries, curl back over the outside of the heart and branch to give a blood supply to all of the heart muscle.

The heart is divided into two halves, right and left, each of which has two chambers, an upper and a lower, called an atrium and a ventricle. Blood is collected from all over the body by the large veins which run into the right atrium. The blood is pumped into the right ventricle, and then pumped through the lungs where it picks up a fresh supply of oxygen; it goes back to the left atrium, through into the left ventricle and is pumped out into the aorta to start its journey round the body again, taking oxygen and nourishment to all parts.

*Ischaemia*

In much the same way that a kettle that is in constant use gets furred up, so do the coronary arteries in some people get blocked. There are lots of theories as to why this affects some people more than others. It is thought that it is something to do with diet, and animal fats have been blamed. Mental tension has something to do with it, and the amount of exercise taken, but the evidence is conflicting and no completely satisfactory explanation has yet been given. If the hole down the middle of the artery gets narrowed too much there comes a time when the heart is called on to do more work than it is getting nourishment for, and this results in pain in the chest, called angina. The pain sometimes goes into the left arm and gives a choking sensation in the throat. If the person stops what he is doing and gives the heart a chance to catch up with itself, the pain goes away. This temporary nature is an important characteristic of angina which helps to distinguish it from a full-blown coronary. It is important that the patient does not try to overcome the pain by keeping on doing whatever produced it. He must stop and rest completely until the pain goes away. This pain is a warning that an undue strain is being put on the heart and it is a warning that must not be ignored. A patient can have angina for years, having attacks every day, but learn to live with it. The onset of pain in the region of the heart does not mean that all activity must cease, in fact a certain amount of exercise, within the limits that the angina allows, is to be encouraged, since, if all exercise is stopped the patient will probably put on weight and become less fit.

There are small, white tablets called glyceryl trinitrate which may be used to help control angina. An angina sufferer should always carry a supply with him. They are placed under the tongue and allowed to dissolve at the first sign of an attack; all activity should be stopped at the same time. A whole tablet may be used or it may be that the pain will subside before the tablet has completely dissolved, in which case the remainder can be spat out. They are very safe tablets and can be used almost without restriction. Some patients need as many as twenty per day and can safely do so without any ill effects, but the average will be considerably less. Some people find they get a thick head after their use. This is slightly unpleasant, but of no serious significance. There is an older type of tablet with a chocolate colour made of the same glyceryl trinitrate which is chewed instead of being dissolved, but the small white ones are much more common.

Some people use a tablet before doing a certain activity they know from past experience will produce pain, in order to prevent it. It may be that going upstairs or climbing a certain hill is known to produce pain; if so, it is quite in order to put a tablet under the tongue as a preventative.

There are other tablets used in the control of angina. There is a group which acts in the same way as glyceryl trinitrate but for a longer time, such that the patient always has a certain amount of the drug in his system. A newer group of drugs stop the heart from becoming too active and can give dramatic benefit to some angina sufferers. They are called B-blockers for technical reasons.

### *Coronary thrombosis*

The words coronary thrombosis indicate the formation of a clot or thrombosis in the coronary artery. This cuts off the blood supply completely to a section of the heart muscle and, depending on whether the clot is in one of the main coronary arteries or one of the smaller branches, a large or small section of muscle is denied its nourishment. The rest of the heart muscle then has to take over the function of the damaged part, which slowly heals into scar tissue.

This can present in a whole spectrun of different ways, from the man who claps his hand to his chest, falls down and expires quickly to the elderly person who feels unwell, but with no pain, and on testing is found to have had a coronary. These are the two extremes, and the average coronary, if there is such a thing, falls somewhere in between. Pain similar to angina in distribution, but longer lasting and more severe, which does not respond quickly to rest or glyceryl trinitrate tablets is the way in which a coronary frequently presents. These patients' prime need is for absolute rest and relief of pain, which a doctor will often give by injections. Most deaths occur in the first few hours, and if the victim survives the first twenty-four hours, his chances of survival very rapidly improve.

During the early period after a coronary there is the possibility of dangerous irregularities in the heart beat which, if promptly treated, can be controlled; for this reason patients are frequently admitted to hospital where their heart function can be monitored and action taken quickly if required. Not all patients are admitted though, and old people especially are often nursed at home.

The aims of nursing in the coronary patient are to relieve him from all unnecessary effort, both physical and mental. Relief of tension should be aimed at from the word "go" in looking after such patients. Reassurance and a calm, unhurried attitude on the part of the attendants can do a lot to help the patient who is severely distressed and worried. This is easier said than done, but a real effort should be made to impart a sense of optimism, which may not always be truly felt, as the sight of a relative in very real pain and danger is not easily overcome. Pain relief will be provided by medical personnel, but it is up to the nursing attendant to help achieve physical rest. In the earlier stages a patient should be confined completely to bed and encouraged to move as little and as gently as possible. There is the temptation for a person who has always been fit and who suddenly finds himself severely ill to try to sit up, rearrange his pillows, etc., in a fairly vigorous fashion in an effort to persuade onlookers and himself that he is not all that ill. This should be gently discouraged. The patient should be washed by his attendant early on, and even fed by hand in severely ill patients. The advice of the doctor should be sought about using bed-pans. Except in the most severely ill patients the doctor will often allow the use of a bedside commode as the effort involved in getting on and off is not great if helped, and balancing on a bed-pan can be a difficult operation which sometimes takes more actual physical effort than getting on a commode.

The diet should be light, with the avoidance of too much fat, and salt should be kept to a minimum. It should be taken in small quantities at a time, and fluids taken between meals, so that the stomach and intestines do not become overfull as this diverts a lot of blood to the intestines, putting a greater strain on the heart.

The length of time that a patient's activities are restricted varies from six weeks' (or so) strict bed rest in patients who have had a major coronary, to an old person who has had a mild coronary and whose normal activities are slow and do not involve great physical strain being back to normal activity in two or three weeks. The return to activity must be carefully graded so that there is only a small increase in energy requirements from day to day, and if pain or other signs of distress manifest themselves, there must be readiness to go back a bit or not increase activity for a period.

During this rehabilitation period the damaged heart muscle is healing to a greater or lesser extent. A bit of muscle that has been entirely deprived of its blood supply will gradually be replaced by fibrous scar tissue, which does not contract and relax, but allows the surrounding heart muscle to take over its function. There will be an area of muscle which is only partially deprived of blood supply, and blood vessels from the neighbouring muscle will gradually increase and enlarge until it is able to function normally again. During this time the heart must not be pushed beyond its limits, although the limit increases as days go by. There is a school of thought that encourages exercise early on in an effort to make the undamaged part of the heart as fit as possible, and in old people it is important if the coronary has not been too severe, to get them mobile again as soon as possible to avoid them slipping into a state of stagnation. The doctor will usually map out a programme of the rate of remobilisation, such as half an hour out of bed after three weeks, a full day up after six weeks, out in the car in eight weeks, and back to full activity in three months.

After a coronary the patient is statistically more likely than the average person to have another, and so the whole way of life should be looked at in an effort to reduce the chances. Many people in middle age become overweight and, if so, weight reduction is often advised. Smoking has a deleterious effect on heart blood supply, and should be cut down or stopped. Alcohol in moderation, apart from its weight-giving properties, does not do harm. Activity should be moderated to the extent of avoiding excessive fatigue, but an effort to keep moderately fit should be encouraged. Walking is good exercise, and walking upstairs instead of taking the lift, walking to the next bus stop instead of the one outside one's house, are good ideas. The sort of thing to be avoided is heavy unaccustomed exercise, such as on the first fine day in spring going out and digging over the whole vegetable patch in one session; and the man who once a week plays a vigorous game of squash after a heavy meal and the rest of the week takes no exercise is asking for trouble. Moderation in all things is a good rule of thumb.

*Heart failure*

When the pumping action of the heart is not strong enough to pump the blood around the body sufficiently for normal bodily function, the patient is said to be in heart failure. Heart failure is a symptom of some disease process either in the heart, such as a coronary thrombosis or a heart valve not working properly, such as mitral stenosis (where the mitral valve between the two chambers of the right side of the heart is narrowed), or it can be due to disease outside the heart, such as infection in the lungs. Quite often the heart can keep going with quite severe disease being present, such as mitral stenosis, but if the patient gets a chest infection this is just too much for the heart to cope with, and heart failure ensues.

One of the main features of heart failure is breathlessness, initially on exertion, and as the disease becomes more serious, at rest, especially when lying down. Heart failure patients use four or five pillows, and in the more severe cases are happier sleeping in a chair, where they are propped upright with the legs dependant, which helps to take some of the strain off the heart. The most severe cases get some relief from leaning forward with elbows on a well-padded bed-table.

As the blood is not pumped through the kidneys fast enough, the fluid is not fully excreted, and so tends to build up in the body as swelling. When a patient is up and about, it goes to the lowest part, i.e. the feet and legs, but if confined to bed it collects in the buttocks, lower back and genital region, which can become severely swollen. Since salt helps to keep fluid in the body, a low salt diet should be instituted. Along with fluid collecting in the dependant parts, it also collects in the lungs, giving shortness of breath and bubbly breathing.

The swollen, or oedematous, parts of the body are very prone to bed pressure sores and extra nursing care is required to stop these developing as, once the skin is broken, it is difficult to get it to heal again.

The heart rate speeds up in an effort to catch up with the body's requirements, and although a slight increase in heart rate does push round the blood more efficiently, as it gets faster it does not have time to fill up properly before each contraction, so its speed becomes self defeating.

The prime need in heart failure patients is rest, as the slightest movement puts more strain on the already overburdened heart, so every effort should be made on the attendant's part to cut down movement to the minimum. Even talking is too much effort for a patient in severe heart failure.

*Drugs* Digitalis is a drug traditionally made from foxgloves, the most usual form used at present being Digoxin. Its action is to slow the heart down so that each contraction is more efficient. Old people are often extremely sensitive to it and need very small doses. Overdosage has to be guarded against as it can occur insidiously, the first sign being loss of appetite, nausea and vomiting.

Diuretics are drugs which help the kidneys to excrete fluid more effectively and so get rid of swelling and breathlessness. There is a large range of diuretics which differ in their speed of action, some acting very quickly so that patients have to pass a lot of urine in a few hours. These are probably best given early in the day so that their action is mainly over by the time they go to sleep. Diuretics tend to wash out a lot of potassium along with the fluid, and so the doctor may advise potassium pills to make up for this. Some of the newer diuretics conserve potassium and so added potassium is not needed.

Since heart failure is a symptom of some underlying disease process, drugs for the treatment of other conditions are used in conjunction with the above, such as antibiotics for chest infection and hypotensives to lower high blood pressure which is a frequent cause of heart failure.

When blood is not passing through the lungs in the normal way patients may suffer from lack of oxygen, and extra oxygen from a cylinder may be ordered by the doctor. Oxygen is under very high pressure in the cylinder and a pressure reducing valve and flow regulator is screwed into the top before turning on. Oxygen is then delivered to the patient along a tube to a mask (usually disposable plastic) which fits over the nose and mouth.

Since failure to excrete fluid is part of heart failure, the doctor may ask for a record of how much the patient drinks and how much urine he passes. Allowance is then made for the insensible loss by water vapour in the exhaled air and evaporation from the skin, and from this it can be deduced if the patient's kidneys are excreting sufficient water.

# 12

# *Management of the patient in plaster of paris*

If the two halves of a broken bone are held together without movement between them eventually the bone will mend. The most common way in which this is done is by using plaster of paris cast as a splint. This is most applicable in fractures of limb bones; there are also other methods of holding bones together by the use of stainless steel pins, actually through the bones. Some minor fractures do not need quite such rigid splinting, and ribs, for instance, are kept in position by the unfractured ribs on either side. Some soft tissue injuries, i.e. to muscle or tendon, benefit by complete immobilisation and a plaster of paris (P.O.P.) cast is a convenient way of doing this.

Casts are made from bandages impregnated with P.O.P., which are dipped in water and then moulded round the part to be splinted. For a matter of a few minutes the P.O.P. bandages are malleable, but very shortly they set in much the same way as cement. The operator has to work quickly to get the desired effect as very soon the P.O.P. is set too hard to work. Although it sets quickly, P.O.P. does not acquire its full strength for about 24 hours and so a patient put in plaster is advised not to put any undue strain on the plaster for that period. When in contact with water the P.O.P. undergoes a chemical change and considerable heat is liberated so that the whole cast feels hot for a short while after being made. In busy accident departments in hospitals the people who make casts get a lot of practice and are able to make strong, neat and lightweight plasters. There is considerable skill in making good plasters; ensuring that the layers are well moulded into each other, giving strength, and not using too much plaster to make the cast heavy and ungainly. Just as it is setting the skilful plaster maker polishes the cast to give it a good finish (which provides an inviting surface for autographs!).

It is a good move for hairy patients to be shaved before a cast is applied as otherwise removal can be painful. An inner layer of stockinette is often used between skin and plaster, but it is not essential. The usual practice is to fold one or more plaster bandages lengthways to form slabs which are applied where most strength is wanted, and then further bandages are applied round and round to hold them in place. This gives strength where it is needed, but not too much weight. Felt or sponge padding can be added around the edges of the cast if there are rough bits that stick into the skin. For certain conditions a removable splint is made by applying a back slab and then using ordinary cotton bandages wrapped round and round. When the plaster has dried the bandages are cut away and the back slab, moulded to the desired shape, remains. This can then be held in position by bandages which can be removed so that the limb can be worked, etc. Certain fractures of the leg are able to bear weight and the day after the cast has been put on a weight-bearing rocker is added under the foot, and after a further period when the plaster used to hold it in position has dried, the patient is allowed to put weight on it. If a plaster cracks from rough use, possibly before it has fully dried, an extra slab can be added over the crack and a makeshift repair effected.

In the hours following an injury, the tissue swells. For this reason it is quite common for a plaster to be applied over a lot of soft padding if it is made soon after the injury. Over the course of the next few days, the swelling goes down and the plaster is too loose. It is then removed and a normal unpadded skin-tight plaster is applied.

A limb that is immobilised will probably waste away a bit, as muscles that are not used lose some of their bulk (and their power). This happens surprisingly quickly, and after a plaster has been on for a week or so it will be found to have become loose. This wasting of immobilised muscle has serious consequences when the plaster is finally removed. When a fracture is united and able to stand stress, it is no use to the patient if he does not have the muscle power to use the limb. For this reason physiotherapy is instituted at an early stage to make the patient use the muscles as much as possible. When the plaster is removed, joints which have not been used for a long time will also be stiff, and it will be the physiotherapist's job to increase the range of movement and help regain full function. A lot of the exercises required are easily learnt and can easily be done without supervision once their importance has been explained, but the will to keep at them is not always there and a certain amount of chivvying is in order.

When a patient leaves hospital in a new plaster the main danger is that the tissue under the plaster will swell to an extent that the blood supply is interfered with. The danger signs are that extremities become painful, blue or cold, or swollen. Movement of muscles helps to pump blood along, and so wriggling of toes or fingers that stick out should be encouraged. The best way of encouraging blood to flow is to elevate the part. It is not much use sticking a leg out in a half-hearted fashion on a stool; what is required is for the patient to lie flat, or even head down, and for the leg to be cocked well up so that it is above the level of the rest of the body. In this way gravity will help the blood to flow out of the limb and so reduce swelling. An arm can be suspended in a sling from a bedside stand well above the level of the shoulder. These measures are often instituted as a precaution in limbs that are likely to swell, and if not, at the first sign of any interference with blood supply. However, if rapid improvement does not follow, medical help should be sought as it is quite possible for the blood supply to be cut off entirely, and if this rare but not unknown situation occurs, gangrene would ensue, and the limb would be lost. This all sounds rather unnerving, but as long as the patient leaves hospital with adequate instructions, no harm is likely to occur. Instructions should be written down, as going through the mill of a busy accident unit is bewildering, and verbal instructions are soon forgotten.

Plaster casts are removed by cutting down their length with plaster shears or with a special type of rotary electric saw which, instead of going round, vibrates. The theory is that in contact with the rigid plaster it cuts through but if it goes too deep and hits skin, since the skin has give in it, it will not cut it. It is true that it is perfectly possible to touch one of these saws on to skin with soft tissue underneath and leave no mark, but in practice it is not wise to rely on its supposed non-damaging qualities as quite unpleasant grazes can be made because the skin adheres to the inside of the plaster and does not have as much give in it as normal.

Care must be exercised with the shears in case a piece of skin adheres to the plaster and gets nipped when the plaster is cut. Where possible it is wise to insert something rigid or semi-rigid between the plaster and the skin to make certain they are separate, and act as a guard against the shears or saw. The plaster, once weakened, can be forced open without having to be cut right through or along its whole length.

After the swelling has settled and a non-padded cast has been applied, the surgeon in charge of a fracture will leave it for a few weeks and then the patient will be asked to attend a Fracture Clinic. After three or four weeks a plaster begins to get worn and weak in places, and so at this time it will be removed. The fracture site is re-X-rayed without the plaster and the extent of the healing assessed. A new plaster is then applied and left for a further few weeks, when the same procedure is carried out. For efficient immobilisation of a bone, the joints above and below it are encased in plaster, e.g. if a forearm bone (radius or ulna) is broken, the wrist and elbow will be included in the cast.

Young people heal more quickly than older ones and an average time in plaster for a common non-displaced fracture at the wrist (Colles fracture) in a young adult is six weeks. A child with only a hairline crack visible on X-ray might only be in plaster for three weeks or so. If the fracture was more severe in the first place and part of the bone was displaced to the extent of having to be manipulated back into place (called reduction of a fracture) under anaesthetic, plaster might be needed for a few more weeks. No hard and fast rules can be given as to how long a plaster will be needed, the surgeon will assess each fracture's progress and when he considers enough new bone has grown for the fracture to be stable without plaster, he will allow it to be left off. As an interim measure he may suggest adhesive strapping or crepe bandages as a means of less rigid support before allowing the fracture complete freedom.

Blood supply is the crucial factor in bone healing. A bone where the supply is good will heal quite quickly, but if a piece of bone has its blood supply interrupted, this will delay healing. Freedom from infection is also important and hence a simple or closed fracture, where the skin over the fracture site is intact, heals quickly. The more serious compound or open fracture where the skin is perforated is slower to heal. Bone is susceptible to infection and antibiotics have made a great improvement in the prognosis of open fractures. In the pre-antibiotic days this type of fracture was often fatal.

The third factor is achieving good contact between the two pieces of bone and maintaining them in contact without movement. Failure in any of these aspects of fracture management can lead to non-union of the fracture site.

Some fractures are not easily immobilised by an external plaster cast. The thigh bone (femur) is so deep in a large mass of tissue that an external cast would not exert pressure on it directly, and so a femoral fracture is not immobilised in this way.

A femur is usually immobilised by traction to the lower half of the leg, pulling against the weight of the body. The patient one sees in bed with a mass of pulleys and weights hanging from the foot of his bed is usually suffering from a fracture of the femur, although some spinal conditions are treated in a similar way. A femoral fracture in an otherwise healthy young man requires about three months' traction.

The neck of the femur is a frequent site of fracture in old people who fall on their hips. Again, it is not possible to achieve immobilisation by a plaster cast, and an operation is performed to put a stainless steel pin through the bone. This has the great advantage that the bone is immediately strong enough to take weight and so old people who easily stagnate in bed and become permanently bedridden, can be got up and encouraged to walk within a few days.

The collar bone (clavicle) is not amenable to plaster either and a system of bandaging which pulls the shoulders back, and a sling on the affected side, are the ways in which fractures of this bone are dealt with. This sort of fracture, like the Colles fracture mentioned above, takes about six weeks.

The notion of six weeks' healing of fractures is fairly well known, and a patient with his forearm in plaster for about this time is commonly encountered. It comes as a disappointment to find that the ankle, which one might consider comparable, takes a lot longer. Fractures round the ankle joint are known as Potts fractures (after Sir Percival Potts, who fell from his horse and spent his time in bed writing about the various types of ankle fractures, one of which he had sustained). Undisplaced, a Potts fracture would require about 10 - 12 weeks, but the ankle is a complex joint and if badly fractured might require longer.

*Simple rules for plaster of paris*

1. Report to your doctor if the plaster becomes uncomfortable or if the portion of limb extending beyond the plaster becomes swollen and/or discoloured.
2. A plaster takes 48 hours to harden completely. Patients must stay at rest for these first 48 hours, otherwise the plaster cast can lose its line and jeopardise the satisfactory healing of the broken bone.
3. Keep plasters dry—even a fully dried out one will become soft if you go out walking in the rain with it on, or get into a bath.
4. Patients in plaster of paris should raise the limb for two to three hours a day. When they are resting it the limb, either arm or leg, should be propped up. This uses gravity to help drain blood from the veins in the limb and reduces the chance of swelling taking place within the plaster.
5. If your plaster gets damaged, cracked or softened, always seek advice about having it repaired immediately.

6. The amount of activity that you carry out whilst in plaster of paris should be governed by the instructions from your doctor: for example, with plaster of paris on the leg, find out exactly how much walking you should do or how much you can do in the way of muscular exercise. The severity of breaks in the same bone vary considerably, and the instructions for one patient might not be the instructions for another.

# 13
# *Management of the post-operative case*

Recently there has been a move towards sending people home after operations in hospital much earlier than previously. This does not mean that the home nurse will be called upon to do complicated management of seriously ill patients with tubes going in and out of them. Usually it is just a matter of "doing time"; whereas, formerly, patients stayed in bed in hospital getting back their strength, and often counting the days until they could get home, now it is the custom to let them home as soon as possible, as soon as the immediate post-operative problems are over. In this way expensive and much sought after hospital beds are made vacant sooner, and surgeons are able to get more operations done, and hence shorten the waiting lists. Most of what is required of a home nurse is common sense, with a minimum of knowledge about care of wounds and the complications, to be on the look out for in the convalescent period.

After an abdominal operation the intestines take a few days to settle down. This is particularly so if the operation has involved a lot of manipulation of the intestines. The slow rhythmic contractions of the intestines, called peristalsis, are inhibited temporarily in a condition called paralytic ileus. This means that food and drink do not pass through in the normal way and, if untreated, the stomach would soon be full, producing vomiting. To tide a patient over this critical period they are given a fluid containing essential nutrients via a tube in a vein, and the normal secretions of the stomach are sucked out by another tube. After a few days' rest the normal movements start again and first fluid, and later light food, is given by mouth. This stage will all be finished with by the time a patient comes home as it needs careful supervision. However, the patient should not have heavy meals early on, and since he will not be as active as normal, this does not matter. There may well be some difficulty in re-establishing regular bowel action as well. Hence the convalescent patient needs meals that are smaller than normal, but care should be taken to give adequate roughage to stimulate normal bowel opening. Fresh fruit should play an important part in the diet, especially citrus fruits such as oranges as they are a good source of vitamin C, which promotes rapid healing.

Patients who have had a cholecystostomy (removal of the gall bladder) will find that they are able to tolerate fat again, whereas before their operation they probably have not been able to. Gastrectomy (removal of part of the stomach) patients will find that they are not able to tolerate a large amount of food at any one time as their stomachs are now considerably smaller. Haemomhoidectory (operation for piles) are usually treated initially by having the bowels confined for the first few days to allow a modicum of healing to the anus. Their first bowel action is usually painful and, thereafter, they should be encouraged to have bulk-producing foods as large soft motions are much less trouble than small hard motions.

An old maxim in medicine is "Rest all inflamed parts", and the site of any sort of operation is an inflamed part until healing has occurred. This advice can be extended to the whole patient so that in the convalescent patient rest plays an important part in the recovery stage. Very often the enforced idleness leads people to having a sleep after lunch. This is to be encouraged in moderation, bearing in mind that too much sleeping during the day will probably mean that it is not so easy to get to sleep at night. The doctor may order sedatives over this stage, but the sooner they can be dispensed with, the better. Even if the drugs themselves are not addictive, it is very easy to get into the habit of relying on drugs to get off to sleep.

If a perfectly fit person were to stay in bed for three days, on getting out again he would feel a bit weak on his feet.

Muscle power and, in fact, the actual muscle itself, very quickly wastes away if not used. This is very apparent when a plaster of paris splint is removed. It can be seen that the limb has noticeably reduced in circumference because of the lack of movement. When in hospital, physiotherapists visit the patients and go through a regime of gentle exercises to make sure that all the important muscles are used daily, so that when the time comes for the patient to be mobilised he has not lost too much in the way of muscle. These exercises are very gentle and do not seem particularly important to the patient, but they should be continued on returning home if quick and full return to function is to be achieved. A person who has had an abdominal operation is very likely to stoop so that the operation scar is not stretched. They should be encouraged to stand up straight and pull their shoulders back even if this is uncomfortable to begin with.

*Post-operative complications*

Anaesthetic agents are irritative to the lungs and bronchi. The gases themselves, which are inhaled, irritate and inflame the lungs and the tube that is often put down into the larynx to ensure a good airway during an anaesthetic sets up local irritation in the upper part of the respiratory passages. The irritated lining to the respiratory system is very receptive to germs and so chest infections are common after operations. The condition of the chest before the operation also has a bearing on the likelihood of post-operative chest infections. A person who has recurrent bronchitis every winter or who smokes heavily, is more than usually likely to get chest infections in the post-operative period.

After an operation an abdominal or chest wound makes deep breathing or coughing painful, and so the lungs do not get inflated to the same extent as in normal health; the normal secretions do not get coughed up, and so collect in the lungs. Added to this, the body has more to cope with in promoting healing in the wound, so that it has less resources to concentrate in overcoming infection. Adequate relief of pain enables the patient to breathe deeply, and they should be taught to put their hands over the wound and press when coughing to counteract pressure from inside. This makes coughing less painful and helps to prevent the stitches pulling too tightly, which could tear the wound tissue and delay healing.

Physiotherapists in hospitals teach deep breathing and encourage coughing up of secretions. They thump the chest and encourage coughing with the patient lying first on one side and then the other and, probably most important, lying flat with the foot of the bed raised so that, in turn, each part of the lung is uppermost. In this way secretions drain from the parts of the lung which are usually not emptied by gravity. As soon as it is feasible the patient is encouraged to get out of bed and move around as this helps to dislodge secretions. Smoking should be discouraged in the post-operative period (it is quite a good time to break the habit entirely) and it is unfair on the patient for people to smoke in his presence.

If infection does ensue, evidenced by a rise in temperature and more coughing, the doctor will give antibiotics to counteract it. At this time the postural drainage and ecouragement to cough are more important still.

In the post-operative phase blood can clot in the deep veins of the leg. During the actual operation the blood flow can be hindered for some considerable time by pressure, the patient not being aware of it because of the anaesthetic. In the immediate post-operative period the patient moves his legs relatively little unless encouraged to do so. The blood itself is more liable to clot than normal as the clotting mechanism is more active having been stimulated by the need for the blood to clot in the operation site. During the operation the surgeon will take precautions to see that localised pressure to the legs is kept to a minimum. In the post-operative phase, movement of the legs should be encouraged to keep the blood flowing through the veins. The practice of putting a pillow under the knees to support them, although comfortable to the patient, should be forbidden as it hinders blood flow in the veins.

The danger of blood clotting in the veins, apart from a swollen, painful leg, is that a long length of blood clot can be dislodged from the long vein, travel up the main veins of the trunk, go through the right side of the heart with the blood, and finally lodge in parts of the lungs, where the blood vessels become progressively smaller again, so that the piece of clot can get no further. This is called a pulmonary embolus.

If the piece of clot is very big, it can be a cause of sudden death in the post-operative period. Much more likely though there is the whole range from the patient complaining of chest pain, having a rise in temperature, and there being blood in the sputum. Any of these should bring to mind the possibility of a pulmonary embolus. Sometimes there are signs of blood clotting (calf pain and swelling) before an embolus occurs, or it may be that it only becomes apparent later on. The treatment of the lesser degrees of pulmonary embolus are similar to that of chest infection. The more painful episodes may require pain relief as well. The doctor may also institute anti-coagulant treatment to lessen the clotting.

*Wounds*

After an operation the two sides of a wound are held together by stitches, and a blood clot fills any space between them. Healing occurs by blood cells penetrating the clot and gradually replacing it by scar tissue. If the two sides are held close together there is obviously very little clot and its replacement is a quick and easy process. Absence of infection and lack of movement between the two sides are the other factors which promote rapid healing. Preparation of the skin with antiseptics before the operation, and aseptic technique during it, lessen the chance of infection. Stitches hold the sides together and rest and avoidance of pressure under the wound help to stop movement of the two sides in relation to each other.

To the patient the most obvious stitches are the ones on the outside holding the skin together, but much more important are the internal layers holding the deeper sutures. When an abdominal wound is closed, first the fibrous layer which lines the abdominal cavity (the peritoneum) is closed, and then the various layers of muscle and, lastly, the skin. The deep layers are usually stitched with an absorbable material such as catgut which is absorbed by the body in about ten days or so, by which time sufficient healing has taken place for the wound to hold firm. In some parts where there is going to be a particularly heavy strain, a non-absorbable material is used so that the stitch material stays in position for good. In the midline of the abdomen even steel wire is used and, of course, this never absorbs and the stitches can be felt through the skin for the rest of the patient's life.

Skin stitches are usually removed after about a week or ten days' time. There are various techniques of skin stitches, some are individual stitches which are cut on one side and then withdrawn, or there are ways of doing a continuous stitch which is just cut in one place and then the whole piece of suture material is pulled out. Metal clips are also used. If skin is being grafted and the graft is held in place by stitches, they will be left in place for a longer time. The doctor may remove stitches from one part of a wound where the wound is well healed on one day, and then remove the rest a day or so later. If the tissue of the wound swells after the stitches have been put in, they become tight and pull deeply into the skin and can become semi-buried, making their removal uncomfortable and difficult. Suture material, if left too long, or if infection is present, sets up inflammation and it can be seen that the tissue around the stitches becomes red and angry-looking. The doctor will then have to choose between the benefits of keeping the stitches in to hold the edges together, against the disadvantage of the inflammation caused by them. The absorbable material of the deep stitches sometimes fails to fully absorb, and this sets up inflammation in the deeper layers. Either this process or infection in the wound can set up a wound abscess which is rather like a boil. The wound becomes red, swollen and painful, and probably the patient's temperature will rise. Pus is found, as in a boil, and this will come to a head and discharge on the surface. The doctor will often open the wound slightly and let the pus out earlier than it would have done so by itself. Usually, this having been done, and with the help of antibiotics, the wound then heals again quickly.

If the surgeon thinks that a lot of fluid will collect under the wound, he will leave a drain in. This can be a bit of rubber tubing or corrugated rubber sheeting—anything that keeps an opening to allow the fluid to drain out. The drain can come through the main wound or have a little separate stab wound away from the main wound in a position where it can drain best. The drains are removed after a few days when it is thought fluid will no longer collect.

Infection can invade blood vessels in the wound and cause sudden bleeding. This may be serious and direct pressure should be applied to the wound and medical help sought quickly. The other emergency that can happen with abdominal wounds is for the wound to burst open and the underlying gut to extrude. No attempt should be made to push the gut back in, it should be covered with a clean damp cloth and medical help sought. Both of these occurrences are exceedingly unlikely; most wounds heal quickly and with no trouble.

The surgeon will leave instructions about if and when the dressing should be changed. If the wound is healing well with no discharge, there is no need for routine changes of modern dressing materials.

The dresser should wear a mask to avoid droplets in the breath from spraying on to the wound. This is more important in hospital than in the home as people in hospital are more likely to carry virulent germs in their noses.

The dresser should wash his or her hands thoroughly with soap and water up to the elbows, having got everything ready first. The nails should be kept short and any dirt removed with an orange stick or nail file.

Old dressings should be put in a paper bag and then burnt. The skin should be washed with swabs of cotton wool dipped in antiseptic solution. Care should be taken that the swabs are not used backwards and forwards, one wipe, and then throw away and take a fresh one.

Sterile surgical gauze folded into a pad is the traditional dressing, but there are now available materials which do not adhere to the wound, and when available these should be used. They are, however, costly. Some people are allergic to adhesive tape and there are available alternatives which do not produce allergic reactions so easily. Sellotape will do the job quite well.

*Colostomies*

If the lower bowel is blocked, sometimes as a temporary expedient or in more serious cases as a permanent feature, a piece of bowel is brought to the surface of the abdominal wall and an opening is made as an artificial anus. The end of the piece of bowel stands up in front of the abdominal wall and an adhesive pad with a hole in the centre is stuck into the skin, encircling it. The pad has a rigid ring to which are attached disposable bags. A colostomy belt is used to hold both in position.

Unlike the anus, there can be no muscular control, so faeces are extruded at any time. Since the lower bowel is very concerned with the reabsorption of fluid to make a motion of normal consistency, when part of it is not being used the faeces are more fluid than normal.

After a colostomy has been made the diet has to be carefully built up to produce a normal stool. Care has to be exercised with the amount of green vegetables as these can produce too vigorous an action. Laxatives are seldom needed, stewed fruit or prunes should be sufficient in small quantities. Secretions from the gut can cause soreness of the skin around the colostomy and barrier creams have to be used to prevent this.

Before the patient leaves hospital he has become familiar with the management and control of his colostomy. It will not have completely settled down, however, and there will be much further shrinking and settling down of the skin tissues until the colostomy is just a small manageable hole on the side wall of the abdomen.

There is often some difficulty settling down at home as the family will become involved initially in the care, dressings and changing of colostomy bags, etc. The district nurse will be most helpful in instructing them and helping the patient himself with the management.

Colostomy bags, dressings, strapping, etc., can be obtained on prescription through your doctor.

Once you have accepted the idea of a colostomy and it has settled down and is under control, it is the most minimal handicap. Many people in private and public life through a complete cross section of society live their lives fully and adequately with colostomies. In all cases it has been performed either to relieve a medical condition or as the residue of a more serious operation, in every situation it can only improve the quality and length of life of the patient.

14

# *Management of chronic chest disease*

The management of chronic chest disease requires a special mention of its own as it is perhaps the largest single area where what one could term the old-fashioned home nursing procedures are still carried out.

Patients with chronic lung disease may spend years incapacitated at home, always vulnerable to infection, always short of breath as their damaged lung tissue can only absorb a certain amount of oxygen for the working of the body. Since the introduction of antibiotics, the outlook for people with chronic lung disease has changed markedly. It has caused a much greater expectation of life and the single condition—tuberculosis—has virtually disappeared from this country, most of the sanatoria which were filled prior to the last war having been closed down.

Tuberculosis does still occur from time to time, and most often after an initial period of hospital treatment and investigation. These patients are nursed at home, where they take drug therapy, streptomycin and I.N.A.H. being the main drugs of choice.

If a patient with tuberculosis is being nursed at home, one must take active precautions about hygiene, particularly when there are young children in the house, and, as mode of spread is through sputum, great care must be taken regarding the patient's coughing and spitting. Always take detailed instructions from the doctor or district nurse about what precautions should be taken when somebody is being nursed for tuberculosis in your household and make sure that all contacts are screened, i.e. X-rays and skin tests to see if they have immunity against tuberculosis or have, in fact, been infected by it.

*Chronic bronchitis and emphysema*

In this condition patients who have had long-standing bronchitis lose the elasticity from their lung tissues and may live for many years with their exercise tolerance markedly reduced, and it is to this group I particularly refer.

For the housebound or bedbound patient with chronic bronchitis, one should apply all the procedures listed in Chapter 10. In particular, room temperature is an important factor, and a change in temperature will often precipitate coughing or increased shortness of breath, so patients should be kept either in one room at the same temperature or, if they are moving to another room, for example a bedroom, make sure the bedroom is warm before they enter it.

Since central heating, patients with chronic chest disease are further embarrassed with their breathing, as the air is drier and the ventilation usually poorer, and this makes it much more difficult to bring up sputum.

If central heating is the only form of heat in a house where there is a patient with chronic bronchitis and emphysema, humidifiers, steam, and the sipping of hot drinks will increase the amount of water vapour in the air breathed by the patient. The same applies to children with a chest condition, paticularly croup, where water vapour is an important factor in helping them relieve their distressed breathing.

Patients with chronic bronchitis and emphysema can develop secondary heart disease through the increased effort of having to push blood through their lungs, and both the chest and heart conditions have to be treated simultaneously. Their main drugs will be antibiotics, which will be used to treat exacerbation of infection, diuretics which get rid of excess water from the body (in this case, particularly the lungs), and in some cases digitalis, which will strengthen the muscular contractions of the heart.

The availability of domiciliary oxygen does mean that many patients who, before, would have had to remain in hospital, can now be treated at home. It must be remembered, if you have oxygen in your home, that this is a fire hazard, and a naked flame near it could cause a serious explosion.

The administration of oxygen must be clearly outlined by the district nurse or general practitioner. I do not think it is sufficient to read instructions from a manual and will not give details of the practical management here, as each case has different requirements.

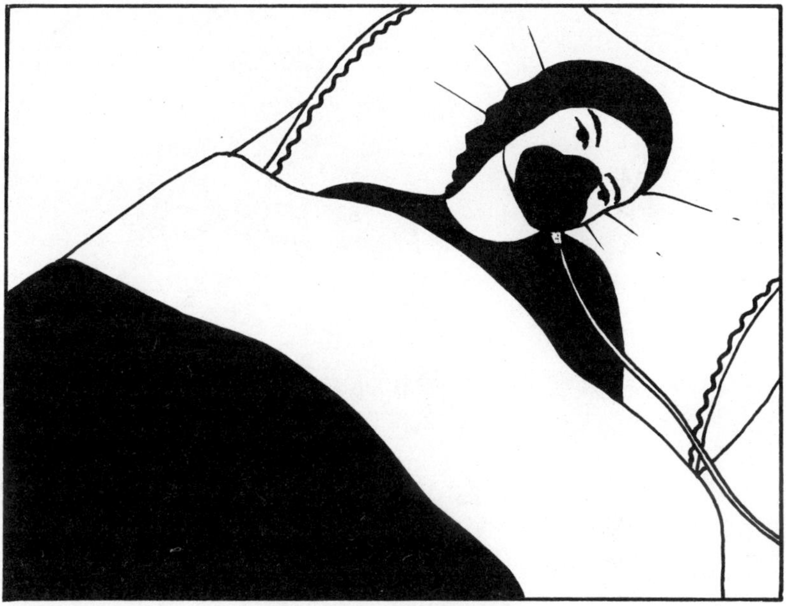

8. Oxygen face mask

There are two main methods for the administration of oxygen, one by facial mask, and the other by nasal tubes.

Some patients may need considerable amounts of oxygen; for example a patient who is fit enough to potter around the house during the day may be enabled to do this by breathing an oxygen mixture thoughout the night. Patients who have lung disease of this severity are under the close care of their general practitioners and the local chest clinic or chest hospital.

Patients who are limited by their breathing ability must learn to conserve what mobile energies they have and use them to the best of their abilities. There are many obvious situations to be considered, such as stairs, access to toilet, distance from living-room to bedroom. Take advice from the occupational therapist to see what aids can be obtained to make the most of a patient's physical abilities. A wheelchair is often forgotten as a means of crossing from one side of

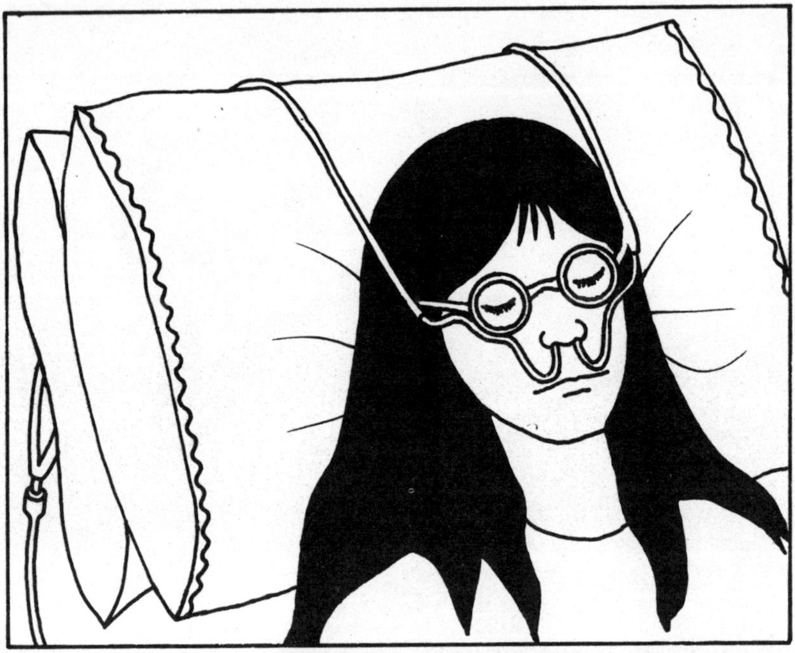

9. Oxygen given by nasal tube

a room to another. When you are expecting somebody who has chronic chest disease home from hospital, in planning which room you will keep him in, take all these factors of constant, even temperature, good ventilation and humidity, access to toilet and bedroom, into consideration and always, when possible, involve the patient as much as you can in the general run of family life. The modern sick-room is not an isolated room with a brass bedstead and a bowl and jug of cold water, but more often a settee in front of the television in the family lounge.

*Smoking*

A definite relationship between cancer of the lung and the smoking of cigarettes has been established. Doctors must warn everybody not to smoke cigarettes. So far the evidence has not incriminated pipe and cigar smokers.

Any rule about smoking that applies to the general public doubly applies to anyone with chronic chest disease. They should not smoke any sort of smoking material at all.

As well as being a related cause of cancer of the lung, smoking is a major factor in the causation and exacerbation of chronic lung disorders.

There is a simple rule for any patient with any form of chest disease — DON'T SMOKE.

*15*

# *Nursing the elderly*

The particular problem of nursing the elderly is that it may fall on the shoulders of one person for a very long period, without any end in the foreseeable future. Often a middle-aged person, whose children have become self-sufficient, will have to bear the majority of the burden of nursing an aged relative, who may not be all that close. Life being what it is, close relatives may be completely committed to bringing up a family or live in unsuitable housing, and so a woman, just at the time she feels she is able to relax after the worries of an adolescent family, will be called upon to take on the duties of nursing an elderly and infirm relative. In more primitive societies where people do not move far away from the family home the burden can be shared around, but in these days where young married couples move away to follow jobs, or in pursuit of housing, the responsibility will often be on one person. This is a part of modern living, which is apparently unavoidable. The State can step in to cover a temporary crisis, it can give all sorts of peripheral aid to make everyday problems easier, but the main responsibility must remain in the family to look after its elderly infirm.

## *Common mental attitudes in the elderly*

It is common experience that a proportion of old people are as "bright as a button" well into their eighties and nineties, and a sharp retort may well come from a centurion. However, some people are "past it" in their sixties and well on the road to senility. No satisfactory explanation as to why some people age more than others has yet been given. Ageing leads to a slowing down of the body's rhythm; old people are content to sit for long periods doing nothing ("soetimes they sits and thinks, and sometimes they just sits"). It is a source of conflict when two or more generations are living in close proximity. The hustle and bustle of a young family can be very trying to old people, and the noise of young children is sometimes more than they can bear. The opposite is also true, that having to control exuberant children in the presence of the old can put an unbearable strain on family life. Hence the old need a place where they can be free from too much going on all the time, i.e. a room they can retire to and call their own. This is not to say that the old should be completely isolated from the young. Watching the progress of grandchildren and getting vicarious pleasure from their vitality is one of the consolations and keenest enjoyments of old age. Therefore contact with more vigorous people should be kept under control, and notice taken when the old begin to tire. Often quiet companionship with slow and not very serious conversation is what is most needed.

In old age the ability to concentrate suffers and an old person who has not had time to cultivate the habit of reading earlier will seldom be able to start late in life. The sphere of interest constricts to the immediate surroundings and a person who has lived a life of wide-ranging interest may become very self-centred and irritable when confined by circumstances to one or two rooms. The television and radio have brought a lot to old people, and now they are able to keep interest going with no great effort on their part. The television can flicker away happily while the viewer "switches off" mentally. If there are defects in the vision which cannot be coped with by the means of normal spectacles the use of a large magnifying glass may help. The public libraries also supply a series of books with specially large print that the old find very useful, but if the sight has gone completely "talking books" are available where the whole of the book is recorded on tape and can be listened to by using the earpiece, and so necessity for reading aloud is obviated.

With the loss of ability to concentrate also memory for recent events can fade. Memory for things that happened long ago in childhood is often retained, and people long dead and occasions long since past are recalled with a surprising wealth of detail; however, this is often coupled with inability to remember the names of people recently met, or what happened yesterday. Mental faculties, however, come and go; there are good days and bad days, and it is quite normal for old people to have two or three days when they seem very senile and feeble, and then recover. These bad patches should be accepted as normal and should not cause undue alarm.

As faculties are reduced by age, of necessity a greater dependance on others encroaches. This lowers morale as the dignity of independence is withdrawn. To have to rely on others to carry out the intimate mechanics of toilet, which in health have always been done in private, saps self respect. This induces timidity in making new contacts and meeting new people, which requires mental effort, is avoided. The daily routine gives a sense of security and hence resistance to change in environment is found. Old people like to be independent and do not like giving up their homes. Normally fastidious people slowly degenerate to living in conditions of appalling squalor, with cold and damp and dirt, but refuse point blank to move to what would seem to be comfortable and convenient homes because it would involve change and loss of independence. This can lead to despair on the part of younger relatives who are not able to give up home and family commitments to go to look after their parents. There are times when this has to be accepted until a crisis such as a broken hip, or even death intervenes. When independence is transferred to another person a very demanding relationship can ensue. A person who cares for the old can find himself bound to them body and soul. Any attempt by the guardian to go out is resisted, and when returning a petulant accusation of neglect is met. This state of affairs should be foreseen and steps taken early on for it to be accepted that the guardian must get away sometimes. A common ruse is for the old person to be "taken queer" or "have a funny turn" if there is the likelihood of the guardian leaving him.

*Promoting and maintaining health*

Every effort should be made to encourage mobility for as long as possible, since the end result of inaction is the pathetic figure with knees drawn up in a fixed position, which makes nursing very difficult indeed, and causes multiple bed sores, which must make the final spark of life a misery. A routine walk after lunch does just as much to aid digestion as a snooze in front of the fire, it broadens the interest, and in leaving the enclosed environment of the house, morale is raised. Too much sleeping during the day, with too little exercise, can well be a precipitating factor in poor sleeping at night. The bowels are more likely to behave themselves if the whole body has had a modicum of exercise. A run in the car is better than nothing—"carriage exercise" it used to be called.

If the bedroom is upstairs and the old person can get up the stairs, as long as it is not causing too much obvious distress no great hurry should be made in bringing sleeping arrangements downstairs as stairs do make a useful form of exercise. In many cases it is obvious, for the sake of all concerned, that life is going to be easier with the bed downstairs, and the above advice should be exercised with common sense. Steep stairs can be dangerous unless adequate hand-holds are provided, and it may very well be a good idea to put in extra hand-holds so that both hands can be used as normal stairs often have only a rail on one side. (Care should be taken that the carpet treads are well fixed, as there can be hazard to the most active of people.) Stairs are often ill-lit, and it is asking a lot of the infirm to go up and down if they cannot see what they are doing.

While on the subject of carpets, rugs that are not fixed, on a slippery floor, can be very dangerous. In the same way that a mother goes around a house and tries to foresee potential hazards for young children and put them right, such as a gate at the top of the stairs, the whole environment which the old are going to occupy should be looked at with a critical eye with the intention of foreseeing where trouble could arise. Many of the safety factors met in a house with young children will be relevant to making a house safe for the old; for instance, care should be taken to use a fireguard at all times. It should be remembered that as physical strength declines, so the ability to react quickly to dangerous situations diminishes. Whereas a younger person automatically is able to correct his or her balance, in the old the reflexes are just not quick enough. Because it is an outward sign that they are not as independent as they would wish, some old people are very unwilling to use a stick with which to help themselves walk. The use of a stick can do a lot to give confidence, the lack of which frequently hinders walking just as much as loss of physical ability; balancing on two points, the feet, is not nearly as easy as when a third point, such as a walking stick, is added. A straight walking stick itself is frequently not sufficiently stable to enable walking to continue, and there are excellent lightweight tripod walking sticks which have the advantage of not falling over if let go. The next stage in progressive failure of mobility is the need for a Zimmer walking frame which can be held by both hands and gives very good stability. Some difficulty in walking can result from loss of muscle power at the ankle and knees and this can be overcome by the use of a specially made boot and callipers which are just struts attached above and below the knee joint to give added strength.

There are also available very lightweight crutches which enable many an old person to maintain the ability to get about. Finally, the wheel-chair is often overlooked as a means of getting some fresh air.

As age increases so does the appetite decrease, in many cases to such an extent that an able-bodied person is often shocked at how little the old need and can be tempted to encourage them to eat more than they really need. This decrease in appetite is not surprising as old people move slower and so use less energy, also their body temperature is lower and 36°C. (97°F.) can be considered normal. When old people neglect themselves and do not eat or keep themselves warm their body temperature can drop even further to a dangerously low level. Every winter old people living alone die from self neglect leading to dangerous hypothermia (low temperature).

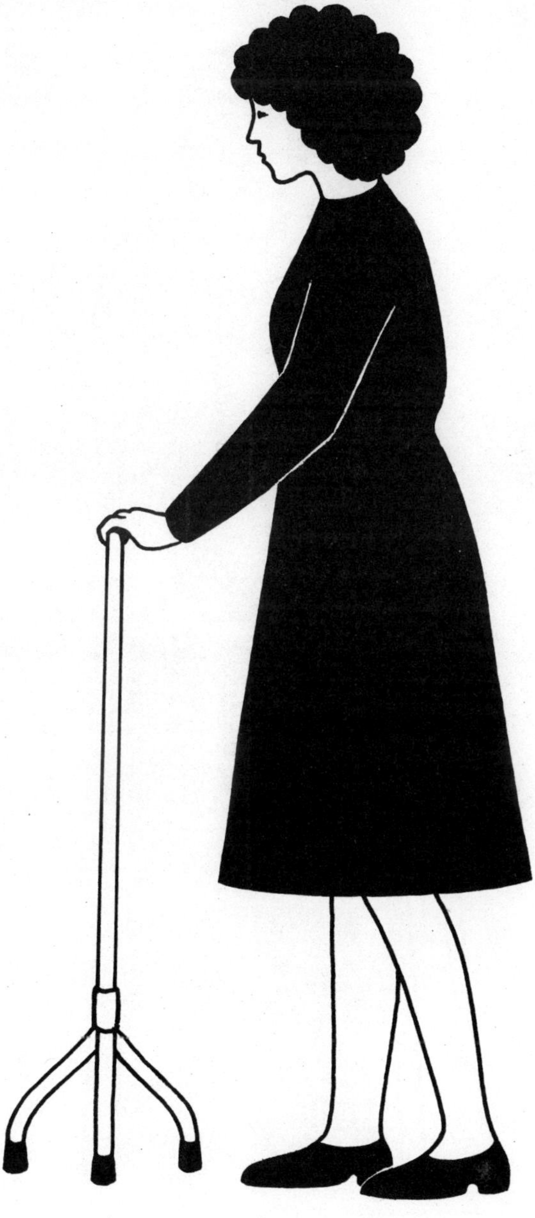

10. A tripod walking stick

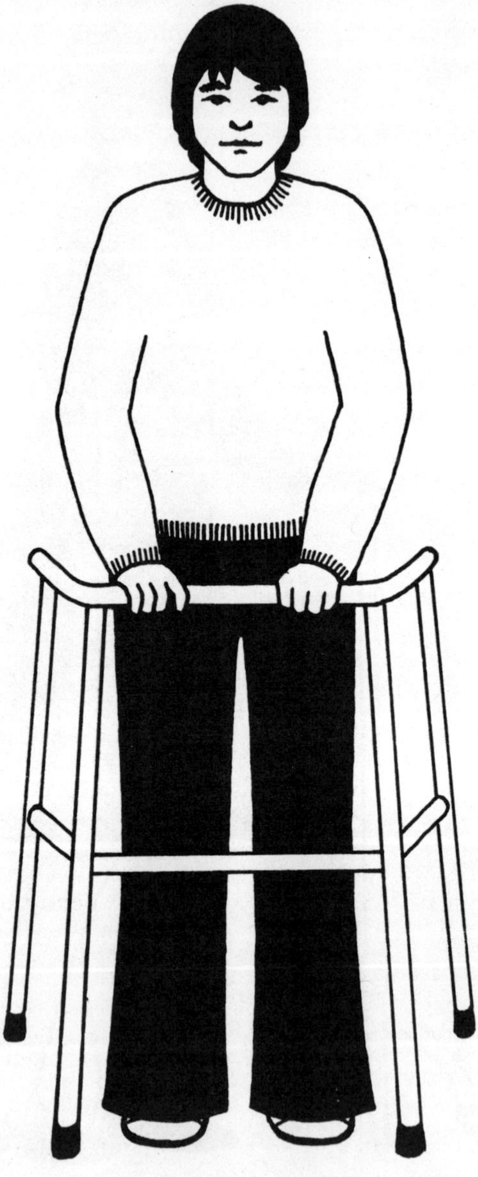

11. Walking frame in use

It is important that the small diet is correctly balanced. Large amounts of carbohydrate (bread, potatoes, cakes and sugar, etc.) are not needed because there is not the requirement of energy for physical work. Some weight loss is quite common and many of the most healthy of old people have obviously "shrunk" from a previous higher weight. Their bodies have adapted to the changing circumstances and requirements. Fresh fruit should be encouraged, and if resistance is met, it is worth having a look at teeth as badly fitting false teeth or maybe broken and rotten teeth make eating an orange almost impossible. A case can be made for giving old people regular vitamin supplements as by the time old age is reached food fads can have become impossible to break and such vitamin deficiency diseases as scurvy are not unknown. Protein (meat, fish, eggs) in regular but not excessive amounts, small quantities of fats (butter, margarine), and diminished carbohydrates is a good guide to old people's diet. This leaves bulk or roughage to be discussed.

Many old people have difficulty with their bowels. They need a long time in the toilet without being rushed by other members of the household. They frequently take large quantities of laxatives, senna being a favourite, and in quantities that would cause extreme discomfort with griping abdominal pain to someone taking them for the first time. However, it may well be that they have been taken for years and the bowel would almost cease to function without them, so it is not a good idea to try to do without them. A lot can be done to keep the bowels regular by adding bulk to the diet in the form of green vegetables as well as the natural laxatives, such as rhubarb. Recently great store has been put by the use of natural bran as available at health food shops. Modern methods of production have removed bran from our flour and bread and it seems sensible to add small quantities—about a desertspoon per day—which can be sprinkled over cornflakes or stewed fruit. This is a much more natural and cheaper way than the use of bulk producers which are available in chemists and which are made from seaweed.

At times the combined resources of diet and laxatives are not sufficient to keep the bowels open. A suppository is the first line of attack which, if unsuccessful, can be followed by enemas. The final method, which should only be used if all else fails, is manual removal, a distasteful job which, nevertheless, has to be resorted to at times. wherby large, impacted masses of faeces have to be removed by hand. A trap for the unwary is to think that diarrhoea is the problem and to give binding medicines containing kaolin. It is quite possible for a person to pass small and frequent amounts of almost fluid matter past a large, impacted constipated mass. "Spurious diarrhoea" this is called, and an enema will often paradoxically put it right.

Old people seem to need considerably less sleep as they grow older and complain of sleepless nights. This is made worse by sleeping too much during the day and not getting enough exercise, by taking too heavy a meal in the evening (for this reason breakfast and midday meals could be made relatively heavier), and by the need to get up to pass water frequently as bladder capacity seems to diminish with age, so fluids should be restricted in the evening. Doctors find in general that old people are difficult to give sleeping medicines to. If a large dose is given, they often get confused and can become disorientated and distressed, also they have a hangover in the morning as their slow rate of metabolism takes a long time to get the drug out of their systems. A small dose is frequently not enough, so simple methods of adequate exercise, and possibly one of the most useful night-time sedatives, a small "night-cap" of whisky or brandy, give the best results.

(It is emphasised that the following is the barest outline, with many simplifications and omissions, and meant only as a guide. Diagnosis must be left to your doctor.)

### *Common ailments in the elderly*

Paralysis from strokes probably calls for more heavy nursing than any other condition apart from plain senility. A stroke means that the blood supply to part of the brain is interrupted, usually by a blood clot, and this in turn leads to paralysis, partial or complete, of the part of the body whose nerve supply comes from the damaged bit of brain. Complete paralysis soon after a stroke may, however, diminish remarkably over the course of the next few months. The merest flicker of movement in a limb can be the sign that significant movement will return in time. Unfortunately a person who has had one stroke is more likely than most to have another, and a series of strokes can occur, leaving increasing weakness after each one. Of course the most distressing aspect of a stroke is if the muscles controlling the bowels or the holding of the urine are paralysed as damage to these leads to incontinence.

Remembering that there is always the hope of return of movement to paralysed limbs, it is important to make certain that joints do not stiffen up through lack of movement and that every effort should be made to stop muscle wasting away from not being used. If, for instance, a leg is paralysed completely, all the joints should be put through a full range of passive movements two or three times per day. In other words, a leg should be lifted up so that the hip is flexed, the leg should be pulled out to the side and then lifted across and over the other, the patients should be rolled over on the side and the leg pulled back and then, putting two hands on the thigh, with the patient lying on his back, the leg should be rolled from side to side. This puts the hip through all the movements that it is capable of. A similar procedure should be adopted for the knee and ankle although there are not quite so many possibilities. The patient should be made to go through all the movements he is capable of and to try to extend the range of movement each time. A patient is quite capable of performing this sort of physiotherapy himself with regard to the arm, using the non-affected arm, and should be encouraged to do so as self help is good for morale and the will to get back function is one of the most potent factors in the eventual amount of recovery.

Many old people complain of a "weak heart" and really are as strong as an ox in this respect, but the signs to look for which indicate heart failure are breathlessness on slight exertion or at rest or on lying flat. Many heart patients have to sleep propped up and the extreme cases are better in a sitting position with the legs dependent as well. A blue colour around the lips and tongue ("cyanosis" doctor will call it) and swelling of the lowest part of the body, the feet in a person who gets up, or over the sacrum in a bedridden patient, are also the principal signs that the heart is not pumping the blood round the body efficiently enough. When the blood supply to the heart muscle is not enough, this produces heart pain, either temporary (angina) or longer lasting, and severe when the blood supply is stopped entirely to part of the heart (coronary thrombosis). People with heart pain must not try to overcome their pain in the way that one might exercise a shoulder to get rid of stiffness. They must rest completely until it is past. Drugs play an important part in the control of heart disease, and patients can end up with a large number of different medicaments.

People who get repeated chest infections usually suffer a certain amount of permanent damage to their chests, and may be breathless and blue similar to heart failure patients. Sometimes there is a mixture of both diseases. They also tend to cough and what they cough up is highly infectious stuff; it should be coughed into a pot or into tissue which can be burnt. The colour is often a guide to whether there is infection present, green or yellow or grey sputum representing infection and colourless sputum being the result of previous damage. We are still dealing with old men who were gassed during the First World War whose chests were permanently damaged and who are particularly susceptible to chest infection.

If a patient is in bed for a long time without moving much and is too feeble to cough sputum up effectively there is a tendency to develop a grumbling infection in the lungs called broncho-pneumonia. Measures to prevent this include keeping the patient as mobile as possible, sitting up, and being given help to cough. It is a common complication in the stage after an operation when there is relative immobility. Whatever other conditions may be present, it frequently is the final cause of death. When someone is progressively becoming weaker, broncho-pneumonia intervenes and puts a stop to suffering, and hence nurses know it as "the old man's friend".

Osteoarthritis is the description given to what happens to

joints from the effects of wear and tear and past injury. The joints get progressively stiff and painful, especially in wet weather, and in the morning before they have had a chance to loosen up. Most old people creak at the joints a bit and a small amount of osteoarthritis is almost inevitable with advancing age. This is often confused in people's minds with rheumatoid arthritis, a condition which usually starts in middle age, whereby the joints get hot and inflamed and painful; it can burn itself out in old age but tends to leave deformed joints.

Cancer is such a multitude of different conditions that it is difficult to give any specific information. In the very old it may be a very slow process so that it is quite possible for a person to die in the meantime of something else.

The prostate gland in men deserves special mention. It is a gland at the base of the bladder which can become enlarged in the sixties or seventies and interferes with the flow of urine. There can be dribbling, difficulty in starting, difficulty in stopping, frequent trips to the toilet to pass small amounts, having to get up frequently at night, and complete blockage with the patient unable to pass water at all. If the patient is fit he is often operated on successfully but if, as is often the case in the old, his chest or heart is too bad he may have to have a tube inserted into the bladder called a catheter which is released at intervals or drains into a bag. The catheter has to be changed at intervals.

Parkinson's Disease affects a number of old people, probably more than is realised, as its early stages can pass as simply due to advancing age. There is a progressive stiffening of the muscles, and movements become increasingly difficult. The characteristic signs are immobile, expressionless face, and "pill rolling" tremor of the hands, that is a constant movement of the thumb and first two fingers as if rolling a small ball. There have been very great advances rcently in the drug treatment of this condition.

Another easily missed condition in women who get fat and lethargic is under-activity of the thyroid gland which controls the rate of metabolism. The signs which make one think of it are thick, coarse skin, thin hair, a croaky voice, and feeling cold all the time (the traditional hypothyroid patient huddles in bed with the bedclothes pulled right over the head and only the tip of the nose showing in an effort to keep warm). This again is a condition which responds well to drugs and is often not recognised by everybody, the doctor included!

### *Incontinence and bed sores*

Incontinence can be brought about by senility and weakness from such conditions as Parkinson's Disease and multiple sclerosis, and from strokes. Usually incontinence of urine comes before incontinence of faeces, or both may come together. Catheters may be used to control urine. With the best care in the world they tend to be messy things, and there is no doubt that introducing a foreign object into the urethra (the tube between the bladder and the exterior) and the bladder tends to lead to urinary infection. However, if they stop the patient lying in a pool of urine, this is a worthwhile disadvantage. Incontinence of faeces makes life difficult for everybody and it is unfortunate but the patients usually manage to get their hands contaminated and hence everything else. This sort of situation is distasteful to the uninitiated, but it can be coped with, and although it could hardly be described an acquired taste, nurses do get used to it and accept it. It is worth bearing in mind that incontinence of faeces may be due to leakage around impacted faeces, and it is not unknown for an enema to give a good clear out and resolve the situation.

Any patient who is immobile for long periods is likely to develop bed sores on the weight-bearing areas. If a part of the body is pressed against a hard surface for a minute or so and then taken away it is seen that, initially, it is white, and then the normal pink colour returns; this is because the blood is expressed out of it. A similar sort of phenomenon occurs when the weight is borne on one area for any length of time, as when a patient lies immobile in bed taking all the weight on certain areas, the skin is denied its nourishment and in a very short time just rots, or more scientifically, goes gangrenous. It is easy to imagine how much more rapidly this occurs if the skin is moist from urine or faeces, and may quickly become infected.

The prevention of bed sores is much more successful than the treatment of an already established one. In a completely immobile and incontinent patient the ideal regime is every two hours to wash the skin over the weight-bearing areas, principally the buttocks, hips, heels and elbows, and sometimes shoulders, and even back of head, with soap and water and, while the hand is still moist, to massage it, using a circular motion. This stimulates the circulation and encourages blood to return to the area. The skin is then dried with a towel, and then lightly dusted, using a non-perfumed talc. Some authorities recommend rubbing with methylated or surgical spirit when the skin is supple and well nourished, but if the skin becomes dry, using a mixture of spirit and olive oil. This has fallen into disrepute in recent years, possibly because at times spirit has been rubbed into open sores if the process has been carried out by young and inexperienced staff. Used with care though, spirit or spirit and oil have a useful place in skin care. After each washing is carried out the patient should be moved so that pressure is taken on a different area. This form of skin care should be started as soon as a patient becomes immobile. If the skin on a pressure area starts to look red, this is a sign that a pressure sore is developing, and special attention should be given to that area and the washing and massage carried out more often. Rubber rings and foam cushions can be used to distribute the weight so that pressure is kept off an area that shows signs of breaking down. Special care must be taken in making the bed to see that there are no wrinkles or crumbs in the bed.

Unshorn sheepskins, woolly side up, have been used in recent years for immobile patients to lie on, and have proved very effective in stopping the onset of pressure sores. Another useful device is the ripple bed, which is rather like a thin inflatable mattress made from plastic but with narrower segments. It is attached to an air pump which sends waves of air pressure through it, so constantly lightly massaging the skin and changing the weight-bearing surface. There is a slight hum from the elecric motor which runs off the ordinary domestic power supply, but patients soon get used to it and find the gentle massaging very soothing. They are much more satisfactory than sheepskin if the patient is incontinent, as they are easier to clean. If the ripple bed is used on top of a plastic-covered mattress, a sheet must be put in between as the two layers of plastic should not be in contact.

The care of skin and prevention of bed sores calls for great perseverance and attention to detail but is of the utmost importance as the treatment of established bed sores is not nearly so satisfactory. The treatment of a bed sore once the skin is broken is to keep pressure off it completely, attend to the surrounding skin as set out above, and to apply antiseptic dressings as ordered by the doctor or a professional nurse. There are many different applications that can be used, and each person has their favourite. When there is a multiplicity of methods it usually means that no one method is entirely satisfactory, and this is certainly true of the treatment of bed sores.

Incontinence of urine is often best dealt with by an indwelling catheter which is a tube in the urethra, with a small balloon on the end inside the bladder which can be filled with water. The balloon stops the catheter from slipping out. The catheter can drain into a receptacle permanently, or have a spigot which is released periodically. The latter is more applicable to patients who have a chance of regaining bladder control as the bladder fills up in the normal fashion and is stretched periodically.

An incontinent patient needs a rubber or plastic draw sheet spread crossways under the buttocks over the top of the normal sheet. This is then covered with a linen draw sheet. Disposable incontinence pads made from absorbent tissue are of great use, and also rolls of the same material, a piece of which can be tucked between the legs and buttock to give added protection. There are also available large squares of material treated with silicone which do not absorb moisture. These are used next to the skin so that moisture goes through and is absorbed in the next layer, hence the skin is never in contact with moist material. Patients can be done up in nappies and plastic pants in the same way as a baby but generally speaking they do not like it and find the plastic pants too hot. Needless to say, as soon as bedding becomes soiled, it must be changed. Lying in contaminated bedding hastens the onset of pressure sores.

### *Outside help*

In nursing the elderly at home various outsiders play a part. The G.P. may call regularly to see how things are going, but G.Ps vary and some may look in when they are in the area or rely on being asked, so that they attend to deal with specific problems. The district nurse often keeps them in touch with the situation and advises when a house call is required.

The district nurse can play a part in calling regularly to help deal with aspects of nursing which require more skilled help, such as the treatment of bed sores, and they and nursing assistants can help with washing, bathing and getting dressed. However, they usually have a regular round of old people to attend to and so can only give help for a limited time for specific problems.

The health visitor has the duty of supervising the general health of the old who are not actually ill and will advise on diet and help liaise with other agencies, such as chiropody. It is difficult to be specific about who does what, as it varies from area to area. The walking aids, and various aids to nursing already mentioned, can be obtained by asking any of these people. In addition there are miscellaneous aids which make life easier, such as rubber mats to put in the bath so that the old person does not slip when getting in and out; handles can be fixed to the side of the bath to give a bit of extra stability. Handles can be put at the head of the bed so that the patients can pull themselves up. In some cases there are sophisticated hoists which can be used so that one person can move a helpless patient.

The geriatric departments of general hospitals often run a system of taking in old people for two weeks or so at a time so that their relatives can get a holiday, and local voluntary agencies may give a relief service so that a bit of free time can be taken. It is important to try to get some sort of relief at an early stage before fatigue sets in. Local old people's associations offer companionship when the patient is still able to get out, and friendships formed at these outings can be of use at a later stage when the old person is confined to the house. A good deal of pushing and encouragement is often needed to introduce old people into these associations.

*Aids for the disabled*

There are many aids available for the disabled and elderly through the offices of the National Health Service. There is no complete list as special infirmities sometimes require specific individual aids. The many standard aids that are available include:

- Tripod sticks (walking sticks);
- Zimmer aids (walking frames);
- Wheel-chairs;
- Bath aids (bars round and across the bath);
- Adaptions to your toilet for raising or lowering, or even ejector seats;
- Hoists and lifting apparatus;
- Bedpans, bottles, commodes;
- Changing of floor gradients to accommodate wheel-chairs;
- Ripple beds;
- Special apparatus for patients who have lost limbs, etc., such as artificial limbs, limb aids, callipers.

Enquiries about aids for the disabled can be made through your general practitioner, district nurse, health visitor, or social worker. They can usually, on demand, quite quickly provide help with such things as tripod sticks, walking aids, wheel-chairs, etc. For the more complex aids that require fitting in your house, it is likely that the occupational therapist will have to visit your home and assess the situation. Here again, the occupational therapist can either be approached through a hospital clinic if you are attending one, or a health visitor, district nurse or general practitioner, as already mentioned.

A great deal of trouble is gone to in this country to provide the fullest help available for disabled people.

16

# *The terminal patient and the unconscious patient*

It is a sad fact that we all have to die sometime, and although everybody knows this, not everybody has come to terms with it fully. The extent to which the fact is acknowledged will affect both the attitude of the patient and those caring for him. If the attendants know that a patient's illness is going to be terminal, and the patient himself does not, an element of deception is involved in any discussion of the illness which can damage the whole relationship. This is not the place to discuss whether a patient should be told, or when, other than to say that a dying patient who knows the truth about his case is easier to talk to than one who does not. The desire to shield the patient from the unpleasant fact is not always in the patient's best interest. It is often because the attendant finds difficulty in facing the truth himself rather than the patient. The fear that an illness could be terminal can be worse than the sure knowledge that it is so. Elaborate attempts to preserve the fiction of eventual recovery in the face of the obvious are seldom worthwhile. Nevertheless, every case is different and a decision about how much to tell can only be made after consideration of the personalities of all concerned and no fixed rules can be laid down.

Despite the prevalence of sudden death in the media, dying can still be an unfamiliar event. The attitude of modern society appears to be that the sight of a dead body should be avoided if possible, and the attitude spills over to cover those about to die. This is in contrast to the custom in less developed societies or in this country a hundred years or so ago, where with a high infant mortality and a scarcity of institutional care for the aged, death was a common family event. Children grew up accustomed to seeing their less fortunate brothers and sisters dying, so that when the time came to look after the dying, there was not quite the feeling of fear and inadequacy which is not uncommon here and now.

When analysed the fear of death is often found to be the fear of the loneliness of dying. A person about to die is a person apart and because of the attitude to their own eventual death there is the danger that those in contact with the dying may build up a barrier which isolates the terminal patient from human contact, leaving him to fight his last battle without the real human contact which gives so much comfort. Unless care is taken to avoid it, the dying patient is talked about in his hearing as if he were not there because, subconsciously, the people close to him are anticipating his death; or whispered conversations are held in such a way that it is obvious that he is being excluded. A person when dying may be desperately anxious to discuss his approaching death but finds a conspiracy of silence surrounding him. This is not a morbid wish to discuss what is inevitable, and if the experience is shared much of the distress can be alleviated.

When it comes to physical suffering, most people think of pain. Certainly some deaths are potentially painful, but pain is a symptom that can be isolated and to a certain extent pain-killing drugs directly combat it and are fairly effective. However, there is the general sense of feeling ill and the discomforts associated with increasing debility which can be the most patent source of suffering to the dying patient.

The occasions on which people are called upon to suffer unbearable, excruciating pain are relatively short-lived and need not necessarily be associated with a life-endangering condition as with renal colic (the pain of a kidney stone passing down to the bladder). The sort of pain that a patient dying of cancer has to bear may not be of such intense severity, but because of its permanent nature and no hope of relief, has a demoralising effect out of proportion to its intensity.

At a certain point in the management of a severely ill person, because of a knowledge of the diagnosis and a combination of an increase in severity of symptoms and general deterioration, it will become apparent to the medical attendant that the illness is terminal. No hard and fast rules can be given about judging when the point is reached, and experience of similar cases is the best guide. Doctors are always wary of giving an indication to relatives of how long a patient is likely to live as a lot seems to depend on the will to live. A desperately ill patient may linger on for months, long after any reasonable expectation, whereas a sudden fatal deterioration over a week or so in a seemingly relatively fit person also occurs. Up to this ill-defined point treatment will probably have been aimed at combating the condition with the hope of slowing its progress or bringing about a remission. This may have involved treatment such as radiotherapy which can itself produce symptoms such as nausea, but it is worthwhile remembering, as experience has shown, that remissions can be brought about. After the realisation that no further worthwhile remission is likely, treatment is aimed at alleviating symptoms. The situation can be complicated by the state of mind of the patient and his relatives. In switching from one mode of treatment to the other it is tacitly understood that there is no more hope. Some people are unable to accept this and it may be necessary for the doctor to continue a line of treatment long after he knows that it can have no beneficial effect, because to withdraw it would have too great a psychological effect.

Drugs which relieve pain are called analgesics, and common examples are aspirin and paracetamol, which are found in many homes for the relief of headaches and other minor symptoms. Although widely used without a doctor's prescription these are effective drugs and in the early stages of a painful condition may be all that is required; for some rheumatic conditions they still remain some of the most effective drugs available. If they are not strong enough the doctor will prescribe more potent ones, but usually trying to use the least powerful drug which is effective so that he has something to fall back on should the pain become more severe. The route by which a drug is given has a bearing on its efficacy, and convenience has to be taken into consideration.

If the drug can be taken in the form of tablets or capsules, this is the easiest for all concerned. However, as a patient gets weaker, he may have difficulty in swallowing and the solid form may have to give way to liquid. Nausea, unfortunately, often plays a part in the symptoms of terminal patients and if this occurs the oral route can become inappropriate. Also, many terminal states involve a slowing down of absorption from the gut, such that even if the drug can be swallowed and retained it is absorbed so slowly into the system that it cannot produce an adequate result.

Should giving drugs by mouth become impossible, the usual practice in this country is to give an intra-muscular injection. Occasionally drugs are given by suppositories inserted into the rectum. Drugs given in this way do not go into the stomach and hence cause nausea and they are fairly quickly absorbed into the system from the lining of the rectum. This way of giving drugs is more popular in Continental Europe than here, but it is used for some drugs in the control of rheumatic conditions.

If intra-muscular injection is used there are several drawbacks. It is, of course, unpleasant to have a needle stuck in, and in severely ill patients who have lost a lot of weight there can be a very real problem of finding enough flesh in the shoulders, buttocks and thighs to give repeated injections. There is also the problem of who should give the injection. They are usually given by trained personnel such as doctors or nurses, but these people are not always available at the time that an injection is required. A person with no previous medical experience can fairly easily be trained though. No great skill is required, just a modicum of common sense, but many people shrink from the idea of pushing a needle into a fellow human being in cold blood.

Practising to use a syringe should only be undertaken with the agreement of the doctor. Syringes and needles now are usually disposable and are supplied in a plastic envelope or case. In this state they are sterile but once the seal is broken they should be used in a short time. Care is taken not to touch the nozzle of the syringe or the metal part of the needle. The drug to be used is sucked up into the syringe by immersing the needle and pulling back on the plunger. Ideally one needle is used to suck up the drug and then it is discarded and another one used to actually give the injection, but this is a wasteful process and as long as care has been taken not to bend over the tip of the needle making it blunt or hook-shaped or to avoid making the needle unsterile, this is not necessary. The syringe is then held with the needle pointing upwards and any air bubble is pushed out. The skin over the injection site is swabbed with a piece of cotton wool dipped in a cleansing agent such as surgical spirit or, more usually now, an individual prepacked sterilising swab. The needle is pushed through the skin, fairly quickly as this is less painful than if done in a hesitant fashion. The plunger is pulled back to make certain that the tip of the needle is not in a blood vessel; if blood comes back into the syringe, it should be removed and a fresh injection made. The contents of the syringe are then pushed into the muscle and the needle withdrawn and the skin wiped over with the swab again. If a bead of blood appears at the injection site, bleeding can usually be quickly controlled by pressing with the swab for a few seconds—occasionally a small temporary dressing is required.

A good way of practising to use a syringe is to inject water into an orange. The orange peel gives a good approximation of the amount of resistance which will be met by the needle going through the skin.

The usual sites for injections are into the deltoid muscle, that is the bulk of muscle just below the point of the shoulder, or into the upper outer quadrant of the buttock, or into the outer or front of the middle of the thigh. These are positions where there are no nerves or large blood vessels which can be damaged by the needle. It is important that no other positions are used without medical advice as there is a very real danger of damaging a major nerve or blood vessel. The point of the needle should be in deep enough to be through a layer of fat under the skin; injections made too shallowly are painful and not well absorbed.

The doctor will start using the smallest dose of the drug that is found to control the pain, but patients may very quickly need a larger dose or the interval at which the drug is given may have to be decreased. Most analgesics, when given by injection, have a duration of action of about four to six hours. Ideally the patient should be kept comfortable and a second one given just as the effects of the previous one are wearing off. The exact timing of this can best be assessed by the person who is in constant contact with the patient and as the disease progresses and the tolerance to the drug increases the normal gap between doses may have to be amended. This is a matter to be discussed with the doctor. The more potent analgesics are drugs of habituation, that is to say that a patient very quickly becomes dependent on them and suffers considerably if they are withdrawn. So doctors prefer to reserve these drugs for terminal cases and, if possible, make do with the less potent drugs in the earlier stages of a disease. The potent analgesics such as morphia, pethidine and heroin are subject to stringent control by law. The drugs must be kept locked up when not in use and a record kept of what is given, in what dosage, at what time, and by whom. Great tolerance is quickly built up to these drugs so that after having received increasing doses over a period of time, a patient is able to take a dose that would be very dangerous if given for the first time.

Although these drugs have provisos about their administration, they are the mainstay of the care of terminal patients in pain, and although due precautions should be observed, a fear of their potency or habituating qualities should be no bar to their being given in adequate doses to ease the distress of seriously ill patients.

When a drug has been given in increasing doses it may be found that further increases have less and less effect and often a combination of drugs is used. Some drugs, such as pethidine, have mainly a pain-relieving function, whereas its close relative, morphia and to a greater extent heroin, although pain-relieving, also induce a sense of well-being and relief of anxiety which makes their use so helpful in terminal cases. Frequently tranquillisers such as chlorpromazine (Largactil) are added to an analgesic and the combination is much more potent than would be supposed from their individual actions.

Good nursing does much to ease suffering. The bed should be remade regularly so that there are no uncomfortable wrinkles under the pressure areas. There is the temptation to avoid disturbing the frail, pathetic figure that a terminal patient can become, but bedclothes in disarray are demoralising and a tidy up is well worthwhile. A regular wash also helps to freshen things up as the skin may become sticky and sour smelling. Special attention should be given to the mouth. A seriously ill patient does not move his tongue and carry out the almost unconscious mouth toilet which those in health do, so that the inside of the mouth can become dry and sticky and the tongue furred. Cleaning the inside of the mouth with swabs of cotton wool, held in forceps and dipped in a cleansing agent such as glycerine or thymol, should be regularly carried out. Male patients benefit from a shave with an electric razor. In short, a wash and brush up which might appear to have no more than a cosmetic effect is beneficial to the patient's well-being.

When patients become bedridden and fail to move about because of general debility there is the danger of bed sores developing on the pressure areas. Regular washing, massaging and avoidance of lying in contaminated or wrinkled bedding, as described in Chapter 15, must be carried out.

When a patient becomes unconscious all his bodily functions have to be supervised by attendants. In normal health breathing is carried out without any conscious effort, but we are only able to do so with a clear airway. If an unconscious patient lies on his back because all his muscles are lacking in tone, the tongue falls backward into the throat and blocks off the passage of air into the larynx and down to the lungs. The outward signs of this are noisy gargling breathing and the colour becoming blue. In the same position anything in the mouth, secretions such as saliva or discharge from the back of the nose, food or vomit, can be inhaled and cause choking. To prevent this unconscious patients are turned on their sides, in which position the tongue falls forward, opening the airway, and anything in the mouth is less likely to be inhaled. A device for applying suction should always be on hand with which to clear the airway of an unconscious patient. This consists of a long thin flexible tube which can be pushed through the mouth or the nose to the back of the throat, and a means of applying suction to it. This may be a simple tube to put in the operator's mouth which connects via a sump, a foot or electrically driven pump. At regular intervals any secretions gathering in the patient's mouth and throat are evacuated.

To facilitate the maintenance of an airway in patients unconscious for a long time an operation of tracheostomy can be performed. A hole is made in the throat below the larynx (Adam's apple) directly into the trachea (upper part of the windpipe) and a tube is inserted to keep the hole open. In this way air passes more directly into the lungs, avoiding the potentially difficult bits at the back of the nose and throat.

If a patient is deeply unconscious, his cough reflex disappears; that is to say, when anything is swallowed, if it goes down the wrong way into the lungs, there is no automatic choking reflex to stop it. This seriously complicates getting any nourishment into the person. A tube has to be passed down the oesaphagus into the stomach via the nose, and liquid can be passed into the stomach in this way. A test has to be made that the tube has gone into the stomach and not into the lungs. This can be done by sucking up liquid from the stomach with a syringe attached to the end of the tube. The fluid from the stomach is acid, and this should be verified by putting a piece of blue litmus paper into it, which will turn red. The other way is to put the tube end into a glass of water and make certain that bubbles don't come out, which is what would happen if the tube were in the lungs. The exact nature of the fluid diet should be discussed with the doctor. The most important aspect is to keep the patient hydrated.

To facilitate nursing the unconscious patient should have a catheter into the bladder so that the passage of urine is controlled. In this way a wet bed is avoided, also the volume of urine can be noted. Since an unconscious patient cannot indicate thirst, the volume of urine is the best guide to the amount of fluid that is required. A normal adult should pass about 1½ litres of urine, and this will require an intake of about 2½ litres as a certain proportion is lost by sweating and as moisture in the breath. If there is a fever this proportion will be raised and a larger intake required.

The bowels also become a problem; if they do not open naturally, suppositories have to be pushed into the rectum, or enemas, and, failing all else, a manual removal.

A daily record of the morning and evening temperature and pulse needs to be kept and, as indicated above, the volume of fluid intake and the volume of urine passed. Notes should also be made of when the bowels are open and what drugs are given.

When a patient who has been ill for some time finally does die it is usually a fairly undramatic event. People do not remain conscious to the last, disposing of their possessions and philosophising until, finally, the head falls to one side, as one would be led to believe in most films. The breathing and pulse are the best guides to the approach of death. The pulse will become weaker so that it is almost impossible to feel before finally ceasing. The breath becomes shallower or sometimes comes in isolated gasps with a few seconds interval, and one does not know whether the next one will come until eventually it is obvious that all is over.

The doctor should be notified when death occurs as he has to certify death: however, if death has been expected there is no great urgency and the doctor will probably have discussed the matter when it is obvious that the end is near. If death occurs suddenly or unexpectedly, nothing must be touched until the doctor comes. The doctor has to give a certificate to state that death occurred from natural causes and also say how long before death he last saw the deceased. At the end of a long illness this is no problem, but with an unexpected death or if the doctor has not seen the patient for more than two weeks, he will be unable to give a death certificate and has to report the death to the Coroner. If the doctor has to report a death, the body should not be moved until permission has been given by the Coroner or, more usually, his deputy, the Coroner's Officer, a policeman. The Coroner may then order a post-mortem examination to determine the cause of death, and can order an inquest before giving permission for burial.

Unless the Coroner is involved, the body should be laid out straight soon after death before the stiffness of rigor mortis sets in. Pillows should be taken away so that the head is at a normal angle, the eyes closed and the chin, which usually gapes open, supported either by tying a bandage under it and over the top of the head or by pushing it up with a pillow on the chest. The main orifices of the body, i.e. the nostrils, anus and vagina in the female, should be plugged with cotton wool and the body should be washed down with soap and water. If desired, most of this can be left to the undertaker. Some undertakers have a day and night service, but there is no great rush, and it is best to take a bit of time to decide how things are to be done. There is no hard and fast rule about whether the body should remain at home or the undertaker should remove it to a chapel of rest, and the relatives are perfectly free to do what they wish about this. If the body is to be cremated, an extra certificate has to be given. The first part of this is filled in by the doctor who has been in attendance, and the second part by an independent doctor from another group, usually a G.P. from a neighbouring practice. The family doctor will arrange this. It is a help to the doctor if the body is not moved until these two parts of the certificate are filled in. With this certificate the undertaker is then able to get authority for a cremation to be performed. The normal death certificate has to be presented to the local registrar of deaths and births in order to register the death. He will be able to give any copies of the certificate that are required for claiming insurance, etc.

# 17 Management of the mentally ill patient

The two main requisites for the management at home of the mentally ill patient are patience and understanding. Mental illness in one form or another is the commonest of all illnesses. This is reflected in that the largest single group of patients who are admitted to medical wards of hospitals are those who have taken an overdose of drugs (self-poisoning).

When we talk in terms of mental illness we have to think of two well-defined groups, one is the mentally retarded, who present in many different forms, inherited conditions, mongolism and retardation due to birth injuries, etc., the other group, what are best called the mental psychiatric patients, suffer from illnesses where the disease affects the personality of the patient in a variety of ways. This group includes psychopaths, schizophrenics, depressives, etc.

For the treatment of mental defectives there is such a wide range of disability that one cannot generalise for treatment and management. The most severe, who cannot cope socially, depending on their degree of disability, may have to live in colonies or in hospitals specially designed for the mentally retarded. Often physical retardation accompanies mental retardation and hospital facilities may be required to cope with the extreme cases of this group.

The less mentally retarded can fit in well into the normal pattern of family and social life. There are many associations which help and advise on the care and welfare of the mentally handicapped, and in most areas there are specific facilities for the mentally handicapped. The emphasis always in the care of the mentally handicapped is when possible to bring them up in a home atmosphere and integrate them into the life of the community as much as possible.

*The mentally ill*

The mentally ill pose a tremendous problem particularly when behaviour is anti-social. In the last two decades the whole approach to the treatment of mental illness has changed. Prior to this time, people with mental illness were incarcerated in hospitals for many years. Since this new approach very few patients are confined to hospital for long periods of time and the day when a doctor, magistrate and psychiatrist certified patients has disappeared. Nowadays if a patient is thought to be a danger to himself or to others and will not take voluntary treatment in hospital, initially he can only be kept in hospital for three days. Unless after this time a further what is known as "Order" is put on him, he can discharge himself, but the psychiatrist of the hospital to which he is admitted can put a further Order on him which covers a period up to 28 days, when the position is reviewed again. Only in a few cases is the third type of Order (which is for one year) applied. This new approach has been a mixed blessing. It has certainly avoided people being kept unjustly in hospital for many years, but it has resulted very often in early discharges where the patient has soon reverted to anti-social behaviour.

Patients who are admitted to hospital with mental illness are followed up at home by both their doctor and the psychiatric worker. Most often in the treatment of mental illness drug therapy is used, and particularly when the patient is at home it is so important that a responsible member of the household takes care of the drugs being given and keeps them away from children. It is important that people acccept that mental illness is an illness just as pneumonia and appendicitis are illnesses, and if they are unable to understand the torments that the patient is going through, these are acutely real to the patient himself. One of the best medicines is listening and all of us are equipped to be able to do this.

Any patient who is mentally ill can be helped by keeping

his physical condition up to standard, seeing that there is an adequate balance of food intake, seeing that they do not neglect their personal hygiene and appearance, and by including them as much as possible into all that goes on within the family. Something like 10 per cent. of the whole population spend some time in a mental hospital. This increases as our longevity increases, as the highest proportion of mental illness is found in the elderly, where part of their illness is associated with the general wear and tear of tissues.

Mental illness is curable like any other type of illness, and people who have had mental illnesses most often are able to return to full communal life, and the fact that they have had treatment for this particular condition does not make them different from other people any more than somebody having had his appendix removed is different.

Every Local Authority has mental welfare officers who will visit patients in the home and give advice and help supervise. There are also many voluntary organisations who do a great deal in assisting with the visiting of patients and carrying out mental welfare.

# 18
# *Services available for home nursing*

If you undertake the long-term nursing of a member of your family at home, that is mainly the care of the elderly sick, do not feel you are alone in your efforts; there is help available under the National Health Service.

1. *District nurses*

A district nurse will be available in the area in which you live to help with the general nursing care of the patient. This includes every aspect of nursing—changing dressings, giving injections, help in the management of patients with diabetes, washing, bathing, exercising and, although laying-out is not included in the duties of a district nurse, where she has become very involved with a case, she will often help with this particular procedure or be able to tell you where such help can be obtained.

2. *Nursing auxiliaries*

Auxiliary nurses assist the district nurse in the carrying out of her duties and do most of the bathing and washing of patients, but do not undertake the more specialised nursing duties.

3. *District midwives*

District midwives attend the pregnant mother both before and after the delivery of her baby. If it is a home confinement, the midwife, with the general practitioner, will conduct the confinement. In some areas district midwives now take their own cases into maternity units to deliver them and return the same day with the patient to her home. She will take care of the mother and baby for the first ten days after confinement. It is the midwife who will advise on equipment for the nursery, and will pay visits to the expectant mother at home as well as seeing her with the doctor in the ante-natal clinic.

### 4. *Health visitors*

The health visitor takes over the supervision of young babies after the midwife has finished her duties. She will advise on further management of babies, particularly feeding problems, and will be present at infant welfare clinics where babies are taken to be weighed and their general progress assessed. It is there that the immunisation courses are carried out, and immunisation is now available against tetanus, diphtheria, polio, whooping cough, measles and German measles. Smallpox vaccinations, which were routinely carried out on babies, are now left until either the situation arises where there is the possibility of smallpox infection or where a smallpox vaccination certificate is needed for travel abroad. The routine and sequence of injections varies from county to county but most commence at six months with the initial injections against whooping cough, diphtheria, tetanus and polio completed in the first year, to be followed by measles and then, later on in school life, German measles and, when required, vaccination against tuberculosis.

The health visitor will visit any patient at either the patient's or doctor's request and will liaise with the doctor about the general care and well-being of his patients. She is the person to approach for meals on wheels and the chiropodist, and works together with the area occupational therapist who advises on aids for the disabled at home and also helps in arranging occupational therapy where it is thought desirable.

### 5. *Social Services*

The Social Services can also be called upon for economic advice and are most helpful in situations where the home economics do not cater for special invalid diets. It is possible, through your health visitor and the Social Services, to obtain help in such areas as night sitters where an elderly, bedridden patient cannot be left on his own and whose attendant relatives occasionally need a night out.

People who undertake the full-time day and night care of the elderly or sick in their homes are considered for a Home Attendant's Allowance, which gives an income supplement to help them in their duties. Details of this can be obtained through the patient's general practitioner or health visitor.

The medical authorities are most sympathetic in their help to families who look after elderly and infirm relatives and cannot get away on holiday and, if approached early enough, will often take the patient into either hospital or guest-house type of care for two to three weeks, allowing the relatives to have a break.

Where patients have to go to hospital for Out Patients, etc., and they have no transport of their own, if public transport is not easily available, transport can be arranged through the Hospital Car Service either via the hospital or through their general practitioner. This can apply not only for attending hospital but for attending for special investigations such as X-rays and blood tests.

The social worker can in some cases recommend convalescent holidays for patients as part of their treatment if this has been advised by the doctor.

The *Home Help Service* is run by a Home Help organiser for each particular area. Here domestic help will be made available dependant on the inability of the patient to cope for herself or himself. The payment of the home help will depend on the patient's overall income. Enquiries about this service can be made through the general practitioner or the health visitor.

## 19

# First aid, and treatment of home accidents

In the management of home accidents the first thoughts should be on prevention, and if you are going to leave children in a room or above a flight of stairs, always check doors, windows, appliances, fires, etc., to see that they cannot harm themselves. In particular, access to sharp instruments (scissors, knives, etc.) can be so easily overlooked. The second requirement is to have a simple knowledge of first aid. The best way of acquiring this is to attend a course of either St. John's or The Red Cross Society and obtain a first aid certificate. A great number of needless deaths arise each year from there being nobody on the spot to deal with the first aid incident when it arises.

Babies and small children, by virtue of the fact that they are learning to walk and crawl and have not always full possession of their balancing faculties, are prone to tumbles, bumps and scrapes, and if not strictly supervised can come to all sorts of harm. If care is not taken to cover fires, see that boiling pots cannot be knocked over, and dangerous electrical appliances are not left lying about, then serious accidents and injuries can result.

### *Bleeding*

Most bleeding arising from cuts and simple accidents can be stopped by applying direct firm pressure to the bleeding area with a pad of clean material, i.e. a clean folded handkerchief or folded bandage. Once the bleeding has been stopped by pressure, then the whole situation can be assessed. If the cut

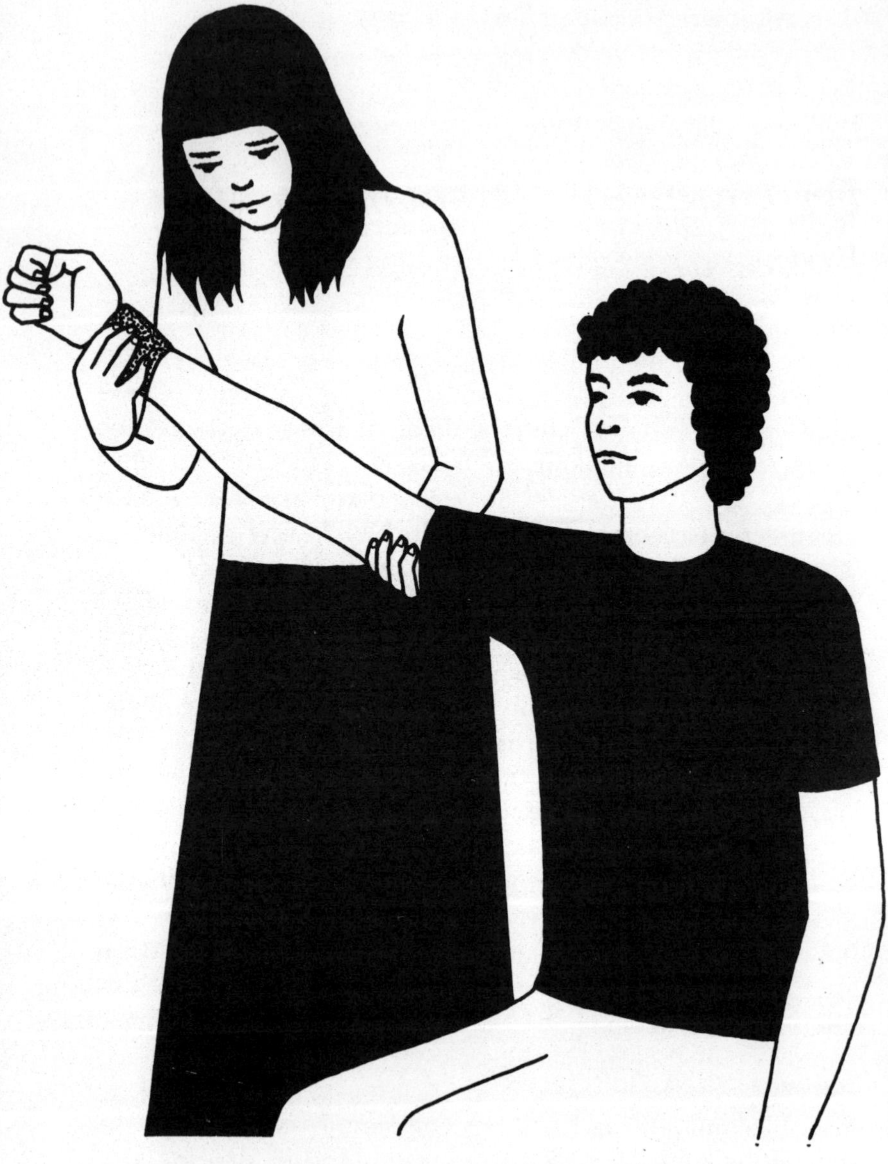

12. Treating bleeding from the arm by elevating the arm and applying a pressure pad

is a large one, it may need stitching, and a doctor's advice will have to be sought. Most small cuts can be controlled by direct pressure. Clean with an antiseptic solution, and dress with either a clean dressing and bandage or an adhesive Elastoplast dressing.

Where bleeding is from the arm or leg, raising the limb means that the blood has to be pumped uphill, and will reduce the flow of blood, making it easier to control the bleeding. Raising the limb alone is sometimes sufficient to stop bleeding. Certainly a cut limb hanging down will encourage bleeding.

*Bleeding from the scalp* The scalp has a very rich blood supply and often a small cut to the scalp can give an impression of tremendous blood loss and a serious injury. It is only on close examination of someone with a scalp injury, who comes in looking as if he is at death's door with a head covered in blood, that it will be found he has only a tiny scratch on the top of his scalp.

Control bleeding from the scalp by direct pressure with a pad. When the bleeding has stopped, clean up with cooled boiled water or dilute weak antiseptic solution and find out exactly what the damage is. If you are in any doubt that it requires further treatment, e.g. stitching, seek medical aid; in the meantime continue to control the bleeding by applying direct pressure with a pad held in the hand, or keep the pad in place with a bandage going round the top of the head and tying under the jaw.

*Nosebleeds* Nosebleeds are extremely common and rarely significant. First, always reassure the patient that nothing terrible is happening. Sit the patient up, head slightly forward, tell him to breathe through the mouth, and grip the soft part of the nose with finger and thumb until the bleeding has stopped. If the patient is old enough, he can co-operate and pinch his nose himself.

Do this for ten minutes and do not let him blow his nose or try to clear his nostrils. If, after this time, he is still bleeding, hold the nose for a further period of fifteen minutes. If, then,

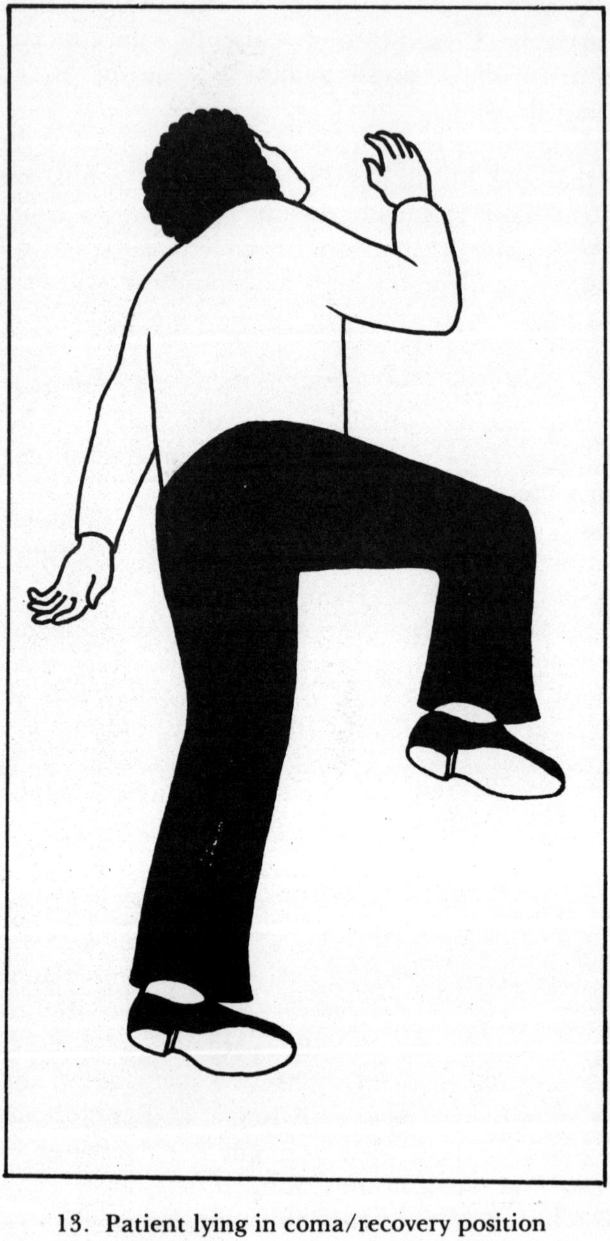

13. Patient lying in coma/recovery position

bleeding persists, plug both nostrils with either ribbon gauze or cotton wool. Unless you are skilled at the procedure, it is difficult to pack the nose of a child. If you are still unhappy about the situation, seek medical aid.

*Bleeding from the ear* If you are certain that the bleeding from the ear is from a superficial cut, treat by the simple procedure of controlling bleeding by pressing directly on it firmly with a pad. Once the bleeding has been controlled, bandage the pad round the head, and seek advice if the cut is extensive and possibly needs stitching.

If there is any bleeding from the ear following a head injury, you must assume that the base of the skull could be broken and must treat accordingly until this has been disproved by X-ray or medical examination. In these circumstances, cover the ear loosely with a pad and lay the patient on his side in what we call the coma/recovery position. This is the position in which patients who have head injuries or who are unconscious should be placed in as it is the position in which they are less likely to come to harm, where a check can be kept on their breathing and where you can make sure that the airway (the mouth) is not blocked by either blood or vomit or foreign bodies.

*Coma/recovery position*

1. Kneel beside the patient and place both his arms close to his body.
2. Turn him gently on his side.
3. Draw up the upper arm until it makes a right angle to the body, and bend the elbow.
4. Draw up the upper leg until the thigh makes a right angle to the body, bend the knee.
5. Draw out the underneath arm gently backwards to bend down clear of the body.
6. Bend the undermost knee slightly.
7. Make certain the head is kept on one side.

*Burns* There is a general principle for the treatment of all burns:

1. Take away from the heat.

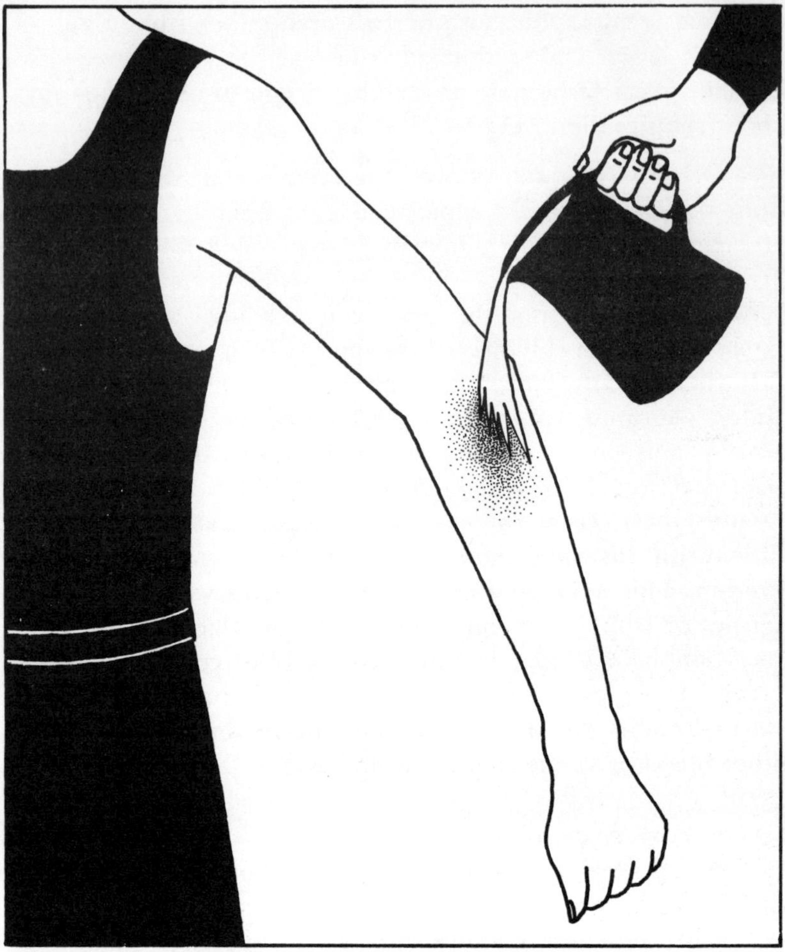

14. Taking the heat out of a burn with water

2. Take the heat away from the burn.
3. Protect from contamination and infection.

This means that you take the patient away from the heat source, pour water over the burnt area, and cover with either sterile or clean material until medical aid can be sought.

For small burns it is sufficient to hold under the cold tap, then cover with clean or sterile material. Do not prick blisters. The ideal covering for burns is Gellanet gauze, which

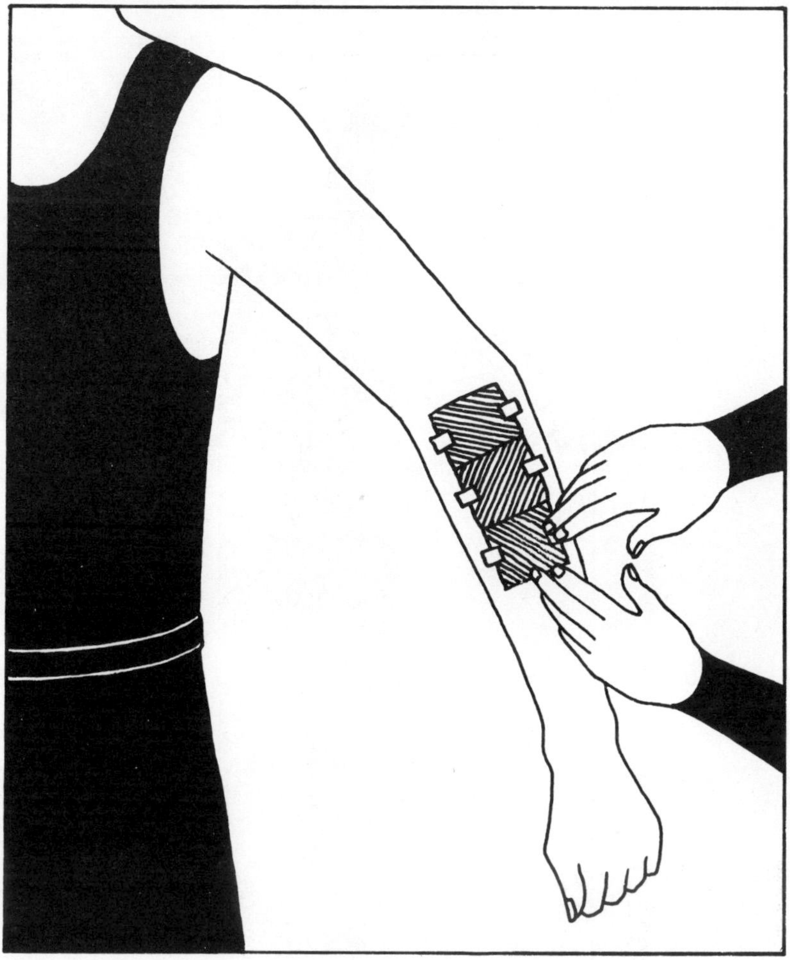

15. Applying dressing to burn

stops dressings sticking to the burn, stops blisters bursting, as well as being soothing. A blister protects the underlying skin and stops infection getting to the burnt area underneath and so should not be burst without medical advice.

Severe burns are a medical emergency. These occur when clothing catches fire, etc., or when inflammable liquids are spilt over clothing or person. The same simple principles for burns apply; for example, if a child's nightdress caught fire the first treatment would be to put out the flames. You do

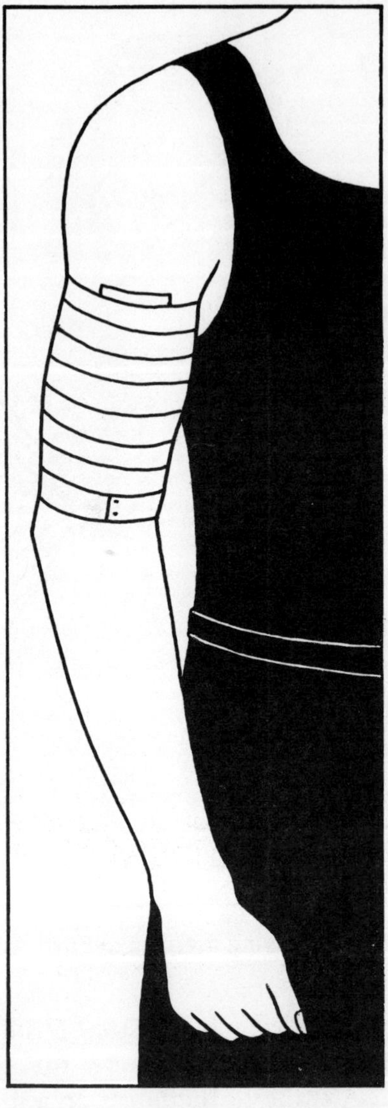

16. Bandaging dressing to arm

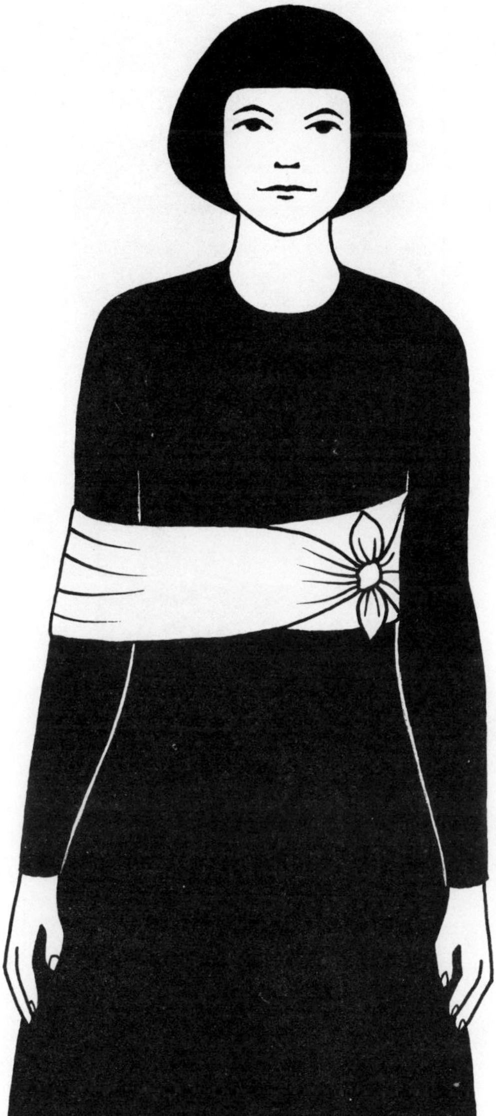

17. Immobilising broken arm by tying to the body

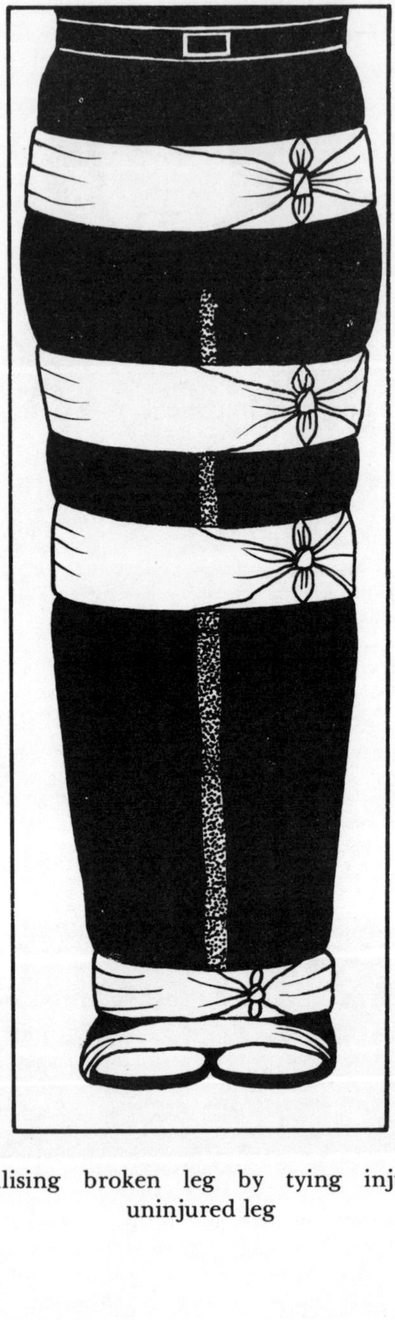

18. Immobilising broken leg by tying injured leg to uninjured leg

this by rolling the patient in a rug or blanket. Take the heat out of the burnt area by pouring cold water over the patient, then wrap in clean material, such as a clean sheet, and take to hospital immediately.

Do not try to remove clothing from burnt areas, but see that there is no constricting clothing such as necks of dresses, belt tops of trousers. Cut through any possible restriction with a pair of scissors before covering and taking to hospital.

*Breaks* Suspect there is a broken bone when a patient has pain in a limb and the limb looks out of shape. The treatment for all breaks is to immobilise, and you immobilise by tying the affected part to a splint, and in most cases the available splint is the body. If someone hurts his upper arm and it looks out of shape, bind the arm to the chest with a crepe bandage, preventing movement of the arm. If there is an injury to the leg, with crepe bandages, with padding between the two legs, tie the injured leg to the uninjured leg, which will make transport much easier and cut down the amount of pain the patient is suffering.

When you suspect that a bone has been broken always seek medical advice as it is likely that an X-ray examination will be required.

### *Common first aid conditions that arise in children*

*Objects in the nose and ears* For foreign bodies, such as beads or insects, in the ear, do not attempt to remove them by probing for them or getting them out on a hairpin. If they do not come out with shaking the head on one side, then they will have to be syringed out by your doctor or nurse.

A great variety of interesting objects can be pushed up the nose or into the ears—seeds, beads, and peas being the commonest. The easiest way to clear the nose is to blow it—don't probe into the nose or into the ears as you haven't the proper instruments and may cause damage. If blowing will not remove the object in the nose, take your child to your doctor or the hospital casualty department.

*Injuries to the eye* For pieces of grit, flies, etc., that get into the eye, try and remove by washing out, that is to say, gently pouring water over the eyeball, with the head on one side and the upper lid pulled up. If the foreign body still remains, it may be gently probed with soft tissue such as a handkerchief. Great care should be taken not to scratch the eye and if there is any resistance, do not attempt to force it out.

For grit and foreign bodies under the eyelids, roll up the upper eyelid over a matchstick or orange stick and flush out with water; then roll the upper eyelid over the lower eyelid.

*Choking* The most important thing when dealing with choking is to keep calm and reassure the child as much as possible. If you can get him to relax he may be able to breathe round his obstruction.

Open the mouth, using something like a spoon handle to get a good view of the back of the mouth, and see if there is something obvious that can be removed. If nothing can be seen, guide your finger gently to the back of the throat and feel for a foreign body. If nothing is found, then more vigorous methods should be applied. In the case of a baby, hold him upside down by his feet. For an older child, place him in the head down position, bang his back and try to get him to cough up the obstructing particle. In extreme cases, mouth-to-mouth resuscitation should be tried without delay.

By far the most important thing is not to panic. Fear is infectious and may prevent practical methods of treatment. Most chokings, if treated calmly, will be resolved by the child coughing or being sick and thus removing the obstruction.

*Fits and convulsions* A convulsion is a frightening experience for a mother to have to cope with. It is important to send for medical help when they occur, although most often the convulsion is over by the time the doctor arrives.

A high temperature often accompanies a convulsion and further convulsions may be prevented by tepid sponging of the baby's body. This will help to reduce the temperature. During a convulsion remove restrictive clothing; check that there is nothing blocking the airway, like food; place the baby on his side so he will not inhale any vomit, and place a blunt object, like a spoon or pen, firmly between his teeth to prevent him biting his tongue. In most convulsions the child will lose consciousness, the body will start to twitch, the eyes roll up and the jaw clench. Persistent fits will have to be investigated, but many children have one or two and don't have any more.

*Drowning*

Your first duties in a case of drowning are: to get the victim from the water; get the water out of him; and ensure that breathing and the heart's action are normal. No time must be lost in starting resuscitation, and in drowning it is worth continuing with resuscitation for up to two hours. Do not cease resuscitation until either breathing has recommenced or a medical expert has said life has ceased.

On removing the victim from the water, place him face down, with the head on one side, and arms stretched above the head. If possible, put in a sloping position with the head at the lowest point.

First raise the body by putting the hands under the stomach of the patient and lift upwards. Ensure that the airway is clear and that the mouth is not blocked by vomit or other extraneous matter such as false teeth, seaweed, weeds, etc. etc. Loosen any restrictive clothing around the neck and waist.

The patient should then be laid on his face with his hands folded across in front of the head, face turned to one side. Then give him a hard thump with the flat of the palm in the middle of the back. This can help dislodge obstructions, restart the heart or even stimulate respiration.

Then kneel on one side of the patient facing his head, the hands are placed under the small of the back of the lower ribs, then you sit back so as not to put your body weight on the chest, then your body is slowly swung forward from the knees, keeping the arms straight and the hands in position, all the time maintaining a steady pressure. Keep this pressure on for two seconds and then relax. A rhythmical pressure is then established in the following sequence:

1. Swing forward.

2. Apply pressure.
3. Release pressure.
4. Rest back with pressure off.

*Resuscitation*

For the unconscious patient where there is no sign of breathing and where the heart may or may not have stopped beating for whatever the cause, resuscitation must be started immediately. There are several methods of resuscitation, one as already described in the treatment of drowning, and one of the other common methods practised is mouth-to-mouth resuscitation.

In commencing any form of resuscitation the first step always is to see that the main airway is patent, i.e. that the mouth is not blocked with false teeth, vomit, saliva, etc., and this must be cleared out before resuscitation can commence.

The principal aim is to put air into the lungs when the patient is unable to do this himself and stimulate the heart to start it beating again if it has stopped. Failure of respiration (breathing) is noted by cessation of movement of the chest and bluish discolouration of the lips, fingers, ears and other peripheral parts of the body.

*Mouth-to-mouth resuscitation* Lay the patient on his back, ensure that the airway is patent by cleaning the mouth. Loosen clothing at the neck and waist. Support the nape of the neck and press top of the head so that it is tilted backwards, pushing the chin upwards. If the patient does not start to breathe, with the chin still pushed up and the head tilted backward, pinch the nose, take a deep breath, seal your lips round the patient's mouth, blow into the lungs and watch the chest rise, stop blowing when the chest has risen, remove your mouth and watch chest fall. This can be continued at the normal rate of breathing until breathing is restored.

In the resuscitation of infants and small children it is important to remember to blow very gently, or damage can be done.

If the patient's heart is not beating, strike the chest smartly

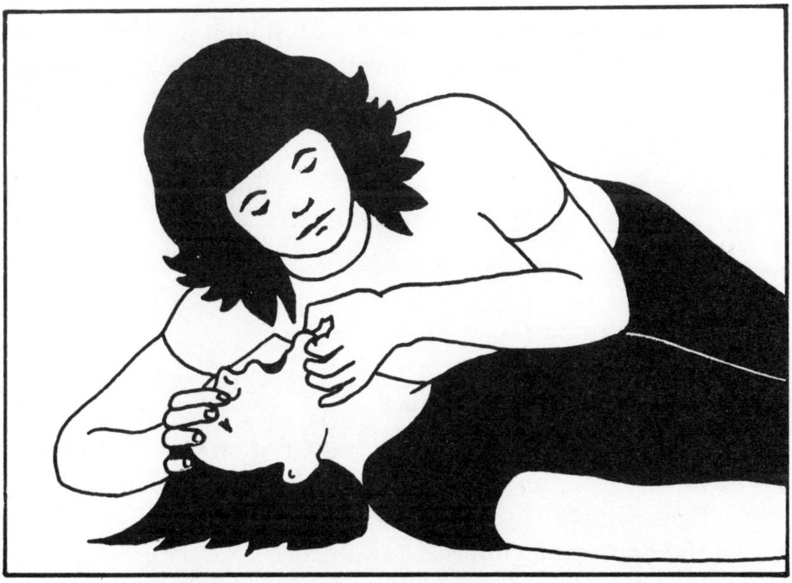

19 & 20. Mouth-to-mouth resuscitation
19. Attendant gripping the nose and lifting chin, tilting the head slightly backwards

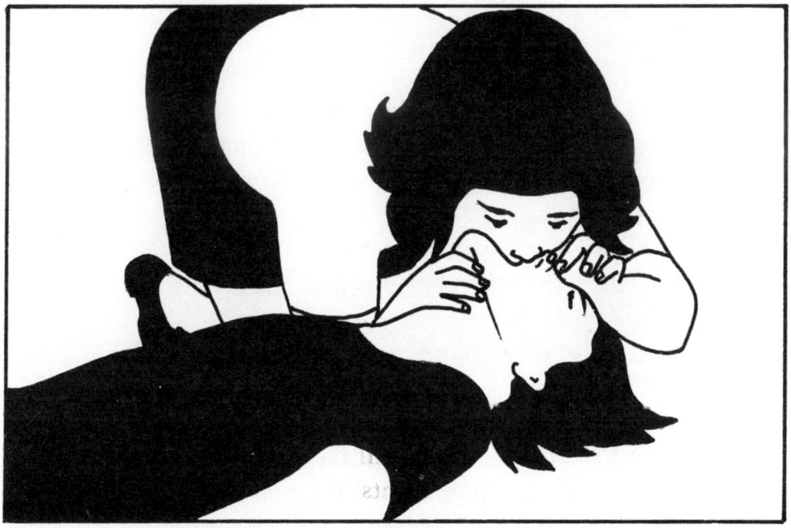

20. With chin tilted and nose gripped, attendant blowing into the mouth of the patient

on the left lower part of the breast bone; if there is no response, start striking rhythmically every ten seconds whilst feeling the pulse.

### *SHOCK*

*Signs and symptoms*

Blanching of the face.
Sweating.
Blurring of vision.
Feeling of giddiness.
Rapid shallow breathing.
Anxious, stunned appearance.
Initial increase in pulse rate followed by weak thready pulse.

*Treatment*

1. Reassure patient.
2. Make as comfortable as possible.
3. Warm, without over-heating.
4. Ascertain cause of shock. See if any local remedy such as stopping bleeding from artery.
5. Summon medical aid or get to hospital.
6. Keep check on rate of the pulse and the rate that the patient is breathing.

### *POISONING*

1. Do not put poisonous substances into bottles with different labels, e.g. weed killer in a lemonade bottle.
2. If the patient is unconscious, move to hospital with all possible speed.
3. If possible, send sample of poison that has been taken. If the patient has vomited, send the vomit with the patient to hospital for analysis.
4. If the patient is conscious and there is no sign of burning around the mouth, induce to vomit by either putting fingers down throat, or drinking large quantities of salt water. Send to hospital immediately.
5. If poisoning has caused burning of mouth and lips, do not give anything by mouth, but send to hospital.
6. For gas poisoning, remove from gaseous area, commence artificial respiration as required.

## *FIRST AID CONDITIONS THAT MAY REQUIRE TREATING IN ADULTS*

### *Bleeding*

*Bleeding from varicose veins* It is important to raise the leg and apply pressure both above and below the cut in the vein as varicose veins can bleed from both ends.

*Arterial bleeding* can be recognised by its spurting nature. In some cases a tourniquet will be needed to control arterial bleeding from a limb. Make a loop of material and insert a tablespoon or stick and twist until there is sufficient pressure in the tourniquet to stop the bleeding. Release the tourniquet every twenty minutes until either the bleeding has been controlled or medical help has arrived.

*Points to watch for with cuts*

1. Deep cuts over half an inch long will probably need stitching.
2. When cleaning cuts and abrasions always clean outwards from the wound, taking the sepsis away from the area. Do not clean skin towards the wound.
3. Check for any cuts, particularly if acquired in the country or farmlands, etc., that the patient has been covered for tetanus immunisation.
4. Send for medical aid immediately and, what is most important, reassure and calm the patient.
5. For penetrating wounds of the chest or abdomen, cover the area with a sterile dressing and treat as for internal bleeding. Do not attempt to remove such things as arrows or knives without medical help.

*Internal bleeding* Internal bleeding can be caused either by injury or a blood vessel breaking. The patient is pale, shocked and sweating, with a rapid pulse. Treatment—do not give fluids by mouth. Place in the position of absolute rest, with the body at an angle of 45° to the ground.

## *THE UNCONSCIOUS PATIENT*

*Unconsciousness*

1. Try to ascertain whether this has been caused by a blow or is for some other medical reason.
2. If obvious blow, treat injured area.
3. See that no false teeth or chewing gum are loose in the mouth, and that the breathing airway is not obstructed in any way.
4. Watch the patient's face for colour sign or change of breathing rate: this will indicate there is some obstruction in the breathing.
5. Seek medical aid.
6. If one can be certain that movement will not harm the patient, put in the coma position to aid drainage of saliva, vomit, etc., from mouth.
7. If respiration stops and the patient begins to lose colour, start mouth-to-mouth resuscitation, as already described.

*Concussion* Any unconsciousness following a blow to the head other than fractional loss of consciousness must be treated as a case of concussion. Keep the patient lying down, cushion the head and observe pulse, respiration and level of consciousness until medical help arrives.

## *SNAKE BITE*

The treatment of snake bite.

1. Tie a firm ligature round whichever limb has been bitten, between the bite and the heart. The ligature should not be so tight as to stop blood going to the limb, but should be sufficient to stop blood going back into the body.
2. Reassure the patient and keep him perfectly still. If he has to be transported, he must be carried; do not let him walk or move the affected limb.
3. Transport to hospital as soon as possible for treatment.
4. When possible, kill the offending snake and take with you so that it can be positively identified. (The only poisonous snake in the British Isles is an adder).

Providing these simple first aid precautions are taken, the chances of death from snake bite in this country are almost nil.

### *THE FIRST AID BOX*

However proficient you may be with your first aid knowledge, unless you have the right tools to hand you will be handicapped in the treatment you have to carry out.

It is essential to have a first aid box or first aid equipment in the house. All households should have at least one first aid box, and car drivers are well advised to carry a further first aid kit in their cars.

*The first aid box*, or cabinet, should be clearly marked and kept in a warm, dry place which is easily accessible though out of reach of small children, and known to members of the family.

It should be clearly marked with a Red Cross.

It is better if it is waterproof, but need not necessarily be air-tight, and should have compartments. It should shut with a firm lid or door, so that it cannot be penetrated by damp or insects, and should be childproof.

If it is to be transported, breakable containers should be adequately protected. If possible, containers should be of plastic or metal to reduce chance of breakage.

*The contents of the first aid box* can vary enormously. Certain essentials are required, and to cut down expense, many of the bandages and dressings can be made from discarded clothing material.

The suggested first aid box is:

1. 1 pair scissors.
2. 1 pair tweezers.
3. Torch.
4. Unbreakable bowl that can be boiled.
5. 6 × 1 in. finger bandages.
6. 6 × 2 in. bandages.
7. 6 × 4 in. bandages.
8. 2 × 3 in, crepe bandages.

9. 1 × ½ in. tin zinc oxide plaster.
10. 1 × 3 in. Elastoplast.
11. 1 packet assorted sticking plaster dressings.
12. Tube or bottle of antiseptic lotion.
13. Soluble aspirin, or Paracetamol, for relieving pain.
14. 1 bottle of bicarbonate of soda.
15. Triangular bandages. (These can be made from a 3 ft. square of material, such as an old sheet, by cutting diagonally across from corner to corner, giving four triangular bandages.)
16. Cotton wool.
17. Assorted safety pins.

*Useful extras for the first aid box are:*

1. Sterile pack dressings (attached to bandages and broken open for use).
2. 1 tin 10 × 10 in. Gellonet gauze dressings for burns. (The author feels that these, although relatively expensive, are a very important part of a first aid box.)
3. Assorted splints, preferably inflatable ones.
4. 1 roll of gauze.
5. 1 plastic water bottle.
6. 1 indelible pencil.
7. 1 bottle of old-fashioned smelling salts.

# 20
# *Common conditions*

## *ALLERGIES*

Allergy or over-sensitivity can appear in many forms, in a baby it can begin with an allergy to cow's milk, from which most milk foods are made, and he may have to have a special dried milk or goat's milk. The commonest allergy is probably hay-fever. But allergy may also appear as eczema or asthma.

The important thing with allergies is to be aware of their possible causes. If a child begins to show signs of asthma, eczema or a rash, check that it is not a dog, horse or some foodstuff like eggs, precipitating it. Your doctor will help, and when the cause of the allergy is traced, avoiding it will certainly help to keep the condition under control.

Any unusual rash, or the lumpy swelling that we call urticaria, is most likely to be an allergy. What is important is that you stop coming into contact with the substance that is upsetting you, either the food you are eating or something you are coming into external contact with. Any allergy will be helped by antihistamine tablets, which can be obtained from your doctor, but unless you remove the precipitating factor, you will continue to itch and swell. So examine carefully any change in diet, wearing apparel or washing powder that might be related to an unexplained rash.

## *APPENDICITIS*

Suspect that appendicitis may be present if a member of the household complains of nausea, intitially discomfort of the upper abdomen, progressing to localised pain in the right lower side of the abdomen. The pulse rate will be up, it is likely that the temperature will be up, and there may be vomiting. Any patient showing these symptoms must be seen by a doctor for appendicitis to be confirmed or excluded.

Appendicitis comes under the heading of an Acute Abdomen. An acute abdomen is one in which the painful symptoms that are arising from it require an operation.

### *ACUTE ABDOMEN*

The term "Acute Abdomen" covers a number of conditions, including appendicitis. If you have severe pain in the abdomen and tenderness on touch, with or without vomiting, and possibly diarrhoea, and you are feeling very unwell, then advice must be sought. There are so many different conditions that can give these symptoms that you should not try to make a diagnosis of which particular condition you think it is, just recognise that something serious is going on in the abdomen and that expert medical opinion is required.

The conditions that can cause this situation are gall stones, inflammation of the gall bladder, stones in the kidney, perforation of a gastric ulcer, inflammation of the pancreas, inflammation of the bowel, and gastro-enteritis.

### *BACKACHE* (*LUMBAGO*)

If a friend says he has lumbago you know exactly what he means, but in fact there is no such condition. The word means that you have a pain in the lower region of the spine, and it can be caused by anything from a kick at football to cancer. What your friend means is that he has pain and immobility in the lower region of the back, following muscle or joint strain. Although most backache does arise from the back, it can also be caused by appendicitis, inflammation of the bowel, intra-abdominal bleeding, and rupture of the spleen. It is the usual first symptom of the beginning of labour and miscarriage, and is a prominent symptom of most disorders of the womb.

If undue strain, particularly in the unfit person whose muscles are flabby, is put on the lower part of the spine, on the few vertebrae above where it joins the pelvis, it can lead to pain and loss of mobility of the lower back. If the strain causes some movement of the spine and interferes with the nerves that leave the spine at this point to supply the leg, then pain will pass along that leg, causing what we call sciatica.

This occurs particularly when one of the fluid-filled sacs (discs) that cushion the spaces between each spinal vertebra is moved or ruptured and the term "slipped disc" is a familiar one.

What do you do when you have backache? First, you have to make sure that that which is troubling you from behind is your back—it is no good going to your favourite osteopath when what you really need is your womb removing.

*First aid* There are few back conditions that are not in some way relieved by pain killers, rest and heat. If possible, crawl into a hot bath, then go to bed, making sure you are lying on a firm, flat mattress, and take some simple pain relievers. You stay there until either you improve to the state where mobility is uncomfortable as opposed to painful, or your lack of progress makes you decide to call in medical help.

*Treatment* The range of treatments is extensive, and stretches from bedrest and aspirins to physiotherapy, manipulation, plaster jackets and surgical operation.

New techniques offer increasing amounts of help to the people with chronic back pain and back derangement. It is so important though to have your back trouble adequately assessed by a competent medical overhaul before starting any treatment. This may include examination of the chest and abdomen, with X-rays, an internal examination, and various laboratory investigations.

*Prevention* Keeping generally fit and physically active, with muscles in good tone, is the best way of preventing back trouble. Tired, flabby muscles, exposed to undue strain, are the common cause. There are specific scheduled exercises for improving the general condition of the back. Take care when lifting, however small the object. Don't bend forward or sideways from the waist to lift anything, even if it's only picking up the cat's ball from the floor. Keep your back in a straight upright column, and let your knees do all the bending, and your legs do all the work. When you take exercise, keep fit for the exercise. A game of football once a month without supporting training can do more harm than good. It is the sudden violent use of untrained muscles that causes damage. You don't have to go to a gymnasium to keep fit—regular walking is as good an exercise as any, and there are many other structures that benefit as well as the back.

This is a push-button age, however, and you are thought of as simple if you walk across the sitting-room to change the TV programme when, so easily, for a few pounds, you could buy a button complex and work it from your chair.

As you sit back smoking, flicking through the various channels, criticising our athletes for not getting gold medals at the Olympics, and blaming the Government for the lack of financial support, the muscles and ligaments that support your spine are getting soft and weak, and if you haven't had backache already, it won't be long before you do.

A simple set of scheduled exercises can be learnt that both help to prevent back troubles arising and rehabilitate the painful back, be it slipped disc, muscle tear or joint strain.

If you are unfortunate enough to develop major trouble in your back, then more comprehensive medical treatment is required. If your neighbour has an operation for his bad back, then it doesn't necessarily follow that you need one too. Each case of severe back trouble is a case of its own, and requires individual assessment and treatment, generally operations only being undertaken when the more conservative methods of treatment have failed. The more you rely on a push-button life, the more likely you are to develop a bad back.

### *BRONCHITIS*

Bronchitis differs from ordinary colds and coughs in that the affected patient is ill and listless. He may cough up or vomit green-looking phlegm. He will breathe more rapidly and his breathing may sound rattly. He will run a temperature and may be short of breath. He will require medical attention and probably an antibiotic.

Where there is central, or gas, or electric heating, the atmosphere of the sick-room may be too dry, and this may make breathing more difficult because dryness makes phlegm more sticky. If breathing is difficult and heating is of the dry type, a kettle allowed to boil in the room will add water vapour to the air and make breathing much easier. (See Chapter 13.)

## *CONJUNCTIVITIS OR RED EYES*

Conjunctivitis or red eyes means inflammation of the outer eye. Do not treat this yourself—it could mean anything from a simple inflammation of the eye to damage or ulceration of the eye. It is mildly infectious, and should be seen by your doctor for treatment.

## *CROUP*

Croup is a type of laryngitis where swellings of the lining membrane of the larynx, or spasm of the muscles, cause difficulty in breathing. It occurs most often at night and is usually associated with a cough that sounds like a barking seal.

The immediate treatment is steam. When inhaled, this soothes the tightened muscles and swollen membrane. The quickest way to give steam is to put a towel over your own head, gather up your child and show him how to breathe over the bowl of boiling water. A child, frightened by his own noisy, difficult breathing, will be reluctant to have his head covered and do it alone.

Having overcome the initial attack, make sure that the child's room is not too dry and moistureless. If necessary, a kettle boiling in the room will counteract any over-dryness in the atmosphere.

Some cases of croup are caused by infections and will need antibiotic treatment before they will clear up.

*DIARRHOEA*

Diarrhoea is characterised by frequent bowel movement with the stool being anything from semi-solid to completely fluid. It is a potentially serious condition in babies, and advice should be sought early if it is at all severe. It is important to continue to give plenty of fluid—glucose, water or boiled water—even if there is some vomiting associated with it.

There are many causes of diarrhoea—unbalanced diet, excessive sugar causing frothy motions, teething, or the presence of an infection such as a sore throat or an infected ear. This type of diarrhoea usually responds fairly easily to simple remedies and the treatment of the source of the infection.

In adults simple diarrhoea will usually respond to starvation and water. If this is not sufficient to control it, then simple Kaolin mixtures will settle most cases, but if diarrhoea is not responding to simple treatment then it must—particularly if associated with vomiting—be considered to be gastro-enteritis, where medical help and medication should be obtained.

*EAR INFECTIONS*

Ear infections may appear either as pain in the ear or discharge from the ears. The pain may be associated with tonsillitis, teething or a boil in the outer ear. A discharging ear may be caused by a burst boil in the outer ear or an infection of the middle ear. Painful ears should be looked at by a doctor as they may require antibiotic treatment, and there is no way of telling whether the ear condition is a simple boil or a middle ear infection without a doctor looking into it. Don't put drops of warm oil into the ears to relieve pain—you are simply introducing a non-sterile substance into an already infected area.

*HERNIAS*

The commonest hernias are round the navel. In infancy it is difficult to decide whether a hernia is present, or whether there is just a protruding navel. If the swelling persists after supporting bandages have been tried, and if it becomes worse on coughing or crying, medical advice should be sought. It is likely at a later stage that the muscular weakness around the navel, which causes herniation, will have to be repaired by a small operation.

The other main group are called inguinal hernias and appear as swellings in the groin, sometimes going into and enlarging the scrotum.

This means that the passageway between the layers of muscle from the abdomen to the scrotum has not closed off and the abdominal contents (intestines) can be squeezed down into the area by exercise or crying. The only danger lies in strangulation, when the swelling becomes hard and painful and the patient may vomit and show signs of distress. The soft swellings that come and go do indicate that surgery will be needed at some stage, but this can be arranged at an elected time between surgeon and patient.

Hernias can be controlled by various types of trusses which are available on the National Health Service. These only hold the hernia in position and prevent it getting worse, they do not cure the condition.

### *SHINGLES OR HERPES ZOSTER*

Shingles is characterised by a crop of blistery spots on one side of the body, forming a curving line. For example, if there are some spots at the level of the navel, there are likely to be crops of spots progressing upwards and towards the back of the same side.

It is caused by the chickenpox virus attacking a single nerve root. It is much more common in the elderly and can be extremely painful and very extensive. If it occurs on the face, great care must be taken to see whether the eyes are involved. Simple lotions such as calamine lotion will soothe the painful skin area but the pain will probably be so severe as to require medication from your doctor.

When it affects young people the condition will clear fairly rapidly, but in elderly people the condition can persist for some weeks. It does not endanger life but patients who have it are usually disproportionately depressed. In the acuter stage of the condition, the patient should be kept at rest as activity does seem to prolong the course of the disease.

### TEETHING

Teething is blamed for more childhood ailments than any other single condition. It can start as early as three months and seems to go on for years. It may be associated with high fever and loss of appetite, and convulsions can occur during teething time.

A teething child often has a red cheek, dribbles, and keeps on trying to stuff things in his mouth. If he is unwell, with a temperature, and keeps on crying, make sure that there is no other cause, such as a chest infection, an ear infection, or even a feeding problem. Teething should be the last diagnosis.

Teething pain can be relieved with aspirin and similar products, but be sure the dose is correct for the age of the child. An extra cuddle from mother will also help. Do not use teething powders containing mercury.

### THROAT INFECTIONS

An infected throat is probably the most common childhood ailment and usually means tonsillitis. Look for large red swellings at the back of the throat, a temperature, some soreness in swallowing and possibly pain in the ears. The pain can sometimes be relieved with aspirin, lozenges and plenty of fluid. It is important to be certain that the aspirin dose is not too great for the child's age. If there is no improvement in twenty-four hours it is probable that an antibiotic will be needed.

Repeated throat infections are sometimes an indication for the removal of tonsils. Nowadays this operation is only undertaken after certain positive indications.

### THRUSH

Thrush, or whitemouth, is a common cause for an unsettled baby. The inside of the mouth is covered by a white fungus and it looks as if the baby has his last mouthful of milk stuck to the roof of his mouth; resistant cases may need a course of Nystatin.

A common site for thrush in adult women is the vagina and a whitish vaginal discharge is often an indication that thrush is present. It occurs more commonly after a course of antibiotics and slightly more commonly in patients who are on the Pill. Advice should be sought from your general practitioner as to the treatment and management of the condition. Many women are shy about approaching their general practitioner with a vaginal discharge but, in fact, 60 per cent. of all women have some type of vaginal discharge which is little more than vaginal catarrh and similar to nasal catarrh. It will respond to medication and strict personal hygiene.

### *WORMS*

There are three main types of worms one may come across in children—threadworms, roundworms, and much more rarely, tapeworms. By far the commonest are threadworms which look like a piece of white thread in a child's motion, and cause iritation round the back passage. They can be cured with various types of medicines, but what is important is that while the medicine is being taken a white ointment, prescribed by your doctor, should be smeared around the back passage each night. Worms lay their eggs in this area and, if left untreated, the eggs will cause reinfection after the worms themselves have been eradicated. Most children get threadworms at some stage of their lives.

Roundworms are much larger and look like a pale sister of the common garden worm. They are easily cleared up with one dose of medicine prescribed by your doctor.

Tapeworms are identifed by the segment formation of the body. It is important if a worm is passed, particularly a tapeworm, to save it so that it can properly be identified. The treatment of tapeworms is a hospital matter.

Worms are best avoided by strict hygiene, i.e. don't put fingers in mouth, always wash hands before meals, don't play with dirt and don't make a habit of sharing the dog's delicious dinner!

# 21
# *Journeys without sickness*

Travel sickness hangs over many families like a black cloud and influences very much where they go and, in fact, whether they go away at all.

This is always a soluble problem; it is finding out what suits your own particular family which is the main objective.

If you find a chain hanging down from the back of your car prevents your family, who are usually sick, from being sick, use it. Or if auntie says the only way is to spread newspaper under the seat and this has worked, try it. If you have found something which suits you, stick to it.

It is no great comfort if you are being sick over the side of a boat to know that Nelson was prostrated with sea-sickness for the first few days of every voyage. All it means is that you're in very good company.

Some people's balancing mechanisms are more sensitive than others and undulating motions, be it car, boat or a roundabout at the fair, will cause sickness. Once you have been sick with any form of abnormal undulating motion, the second time you travel this particular way you are halfway to being sick before you start.

First steps in combating travel sickness are to eliminate as much as possible the motion that causes it. Children who are sick will travel better if they are lying down. Adults should settle themselves comfortably with a stream of fresh air and avoid fug or smoke as much as possible.

Stick generally to your normal routine of meals, for the advantages of travelling on an empty stomach will be offset by the fact that you have upset your routine and are already pre-conditioning yourself to being sick. If you have a history of sickness, take some form of travel-sickness tablets. These are best prescribed by your doctor and you should certainly take nothing without consulting him if you are pregnant.

There are many very good commercial preparations which you can buy on the market, but one must remember that most anti-sickness preparations are derived from the drug hyoscine, whose side effects are dryness of the mouth and tendency to make one sleep. So there is a possibility that a travel-sickness tablet might reduce your judgment if you were in charge of a vehicle.

Take all forms of travel-sickness tablets a good hour before starting a journey—it is too late to take them once the journey has started. If you are travelling by sea, take them an hour or two hours before the ship leaves, and if you are not sick the first day don't be too confident—take a tablet the second day and each following morning. It is much easier to prevent sickness coming on than to stop it once it has started.

For car travel, have regular stops every two hours, when you can get out and stretch your legs and go to the lavatory. Avoid reading in a car, because then you are giving your balancing mechansim extra work to do.

There is no need for anybody to be travel sick provided they take the necessary precautions, be it tablets, auntie's remedy or whatever you like.

## 22
# *Hospitals*

A hospital can seem a bewildering and intimidating place to a patient going there for the first time. The wards and corridors are full of uniformed figures in a hurry, but it must be remembered that all this bustle is designed to be for the patient's own welfare. It may all seem very strange to the newcomer but for those who work there, there is an atmosphere of fellowship rather like that in a school or Army regiment. The patient's well-being is the hospital's reason for existence and so the new patient is soon caught up in the momentum of the place and made to feel at home.

It is very expensive indeed for a patient to occupy a bed in hospital and is becoming more so all the time. This is not surprising when one considers the ratio of staff to patients. Not only are there the nurses and doctors that immediately come to mind when one thinks about hospitals, but there has to be a large domestic staff, and porters, numerous physiotherapists, radiologists and occupational therapists, and then the list goes on to include audiologists, pathologists, laboratory technicians, administrators, secretaries, and hospital social workers. The wages of all these people have to be paid as well as the cost of installing and maintaining expensive specialised equipment. Because of the high cost of having a patient in hospital, as much as possible is done from home and as an outpatient. Admission is reserved for those procedures that can only be carried out as an inpatient. The old attitude of "once they get you in there, they'll never let you go" is the opposite of the truth. Waiting lists seem to grow all the time and hospitals try to increase their turnover to cope with this, so the average length of stay in hospital is steadily decreasing.

To become State Registered, nurses undergo a three-year training and are known as First-, Second-, or Third-year Pupil Nurses. Some take a two-year course to become State Enrolled. These are the girls, and of late an increasing number of young men, with whom a patient has most day-to-day contact. After their final exams, State Registered Nurses (SRNs) can take the job of Staff Nurse, who is the second-in-command in a ward and, at a later stage, that of Sister. (The male equivalent is called a Charge Nurse.) There are differences of belts, caps, badges, etc., with which to distinguish the various grades of nurses, but the Sister often has a uniform of a different colour, which makes her stand out. The distinguishing marks vary from hospital to hospital, as do the uniforms. Nurses who want to follow the career right through can go from the stage of looking after a ward to that of having supervision over a particular section of the hospital, and so on.

Since the Salmon Report on the organisation of nursing, titles such as Sister or Matron, etc., have been officially replaced by numbered grades, but the old titles are still in common use.

After qualification doctors take on the job of Houseman. These posts are usually held for six months, and a doctor will do several in different branches of medicine to widen his experience before specialising. The House Physician or House Surgeon is usually the young doctor who is seen most in the everyday running of the wards. As he settles to one specialty, the doctor will move up through the grades of Senior House Officer, Junior and Senior Registrar, during which time he will be studying for the extremely testing post-graduate exams. Having gained his qualifications he can then seek the post of Consultant. The medical staff work together in groups known as Firms, headed by one or more Consultants. Since Consultants often work at more than one hospital, in any one place they may share a Registrar and Houseman. The Consultant sets the standard and method of treatment in a Firm, but the practicalities may well be carried out by the

Registrars and Housemen. Thus, although being admitted nominally under a certain Consultant, it does not necessarily follow that he would personally carry out an operation or order specific treatment, but his general way of doing things would be followed and he carries overall supervision and responsibility.

There is a convention that Surgeons are called Mister, and this covers General Surgeons, Orthopaedics (bone surgery), E.N.T. (ears, nose and throat), gynaecologists (diseases of women) or anybody who carries out operations, as in the more specialised fields of thoracic or plastic surgery. Physicians are concerned with non-operative treatment such as general medicine, rheumatology and geriatrics (the care of the aged), and are called Doctor.

If the need is urgent, admission to hospital can be arranged very quickly indeed. Following road accidents and the like, ambulance personnel take the injured straight to the nearest Accident and Emergency Department (what used to be called "Casualty") where the need for admission is assessed and any immediate treatment carried out. This can be the route for any emergency where it is inappropriate to take the patient home to the family doctor. However, the Accident and Emergency Departments should be reserved for genuine emergencies and not used as an alternative to the family doctor because of convenience. When illness occurs at home the first contact should be to the family doctor. If he thinks admission is needed, he will ring the hospital and speak to the Houseman of the relevant specialty and arrange admission. Usually this is straightforward and the patient can be in hospital just as soon as the transport can be arranged. In some areas where the pressure on beds is high, admissions have to be made through a Bed Bureau which finds an empty bed from a hospital in the area. In complicated cases the G.P. can get a Consultant to come and see the patient at home, a domiciliary visit, at which a decision about admission can be made. In less urgent cases, where the patient is up and about, he may have been seeing the G.P. at his surgery, and the G.P. will organise for the patient to attend the hospital outpatient department. There he will see the Specialist who puts him on his waiting list for admission. Again, the really urgent cases will be admitted quickly, but it is a sad fact that the waiting lists for non-urgent cases such as hernia repairs or stripping of varicose veins can be very long indeed, each new urgent case pushing them further back.

Much investigation can be done on an outpatient basis, initially by the G.P. and later by the Consultant, but if a large number of tests need to be got through in a short time, it can be more convenient to admit the patient for an intensive week of investigation.

Hospitals are starting to run wards on a Monday to Friday basis for this purpose, as it relieves pressure on staff and allows the ward to be closed at the week-end.

It will be seen that the old concept of a hospital as a place of rest is giving way to that of a place where sophisticated procedures can be carried out. Even in geriatrics the emphasis is on rehabilitation and getting an old person who has become temporarily bedridden back on his feet. Where rest is all that is required, this must be either at home or in a less specialised unit than a general hospital, such as a convalescent home. Nevertheless hospitals are still a place of compassion and are directed to the needs of the sick, and part of their work is to care for those who are too sick to be nursed at home and where the nursing care is too great a burden to be borne in the home situation.

When going into hospital in a hurry, it is best to concentrate on essentials in the way of what to take. The minimum should include two sets of night-clothing—cotton is more comfortable in the long run than nylon, and female patients will be wise to take a nightie which is not too revealing! A dressing-gown; pair of slippers; washing and shaving equipment or cosmetics; and something to read to make up the list. Other things can be brought in by visitors at a later date; outdoor clothing need not be brought until near the time for discharge. If, for any reason, things like a dressing-gown are not available, there is no need to worry; hospitals can cope with the absolutely destitute and will provide from store any articles which are missing. If the patient has been on drugs from his G.P., there is no need to take them into hospital. Any drugs given in hospital will be issued by the hospital pharmacy and drugs brought in will not be allowed to be used.

Although there is a growing tendency to do small operations as day patients, that is they come in the morning, have their operation, get over the anaesthetic, and are sent home the same evening without proper overnight admission, for major operations it is usual to admit the day before to allow some preliminaries to be carried out and the patient to become accustomed to the surroundings. A time to attend the hospital will have been notified, and this should be adhered to. If arrival is too late, essential laboratory tests such as blood grouping, may not be able to be completed. If for any reason it is not possible to go in on the date given, the hospital should be informed without delay as it may be possible to get another patient in and so not waste precious bed space.

On arrival at the ward, personal particulars will be taken for the records, and then the patient will be asked to get into bed. This may be in the middle of the day and the patient may be feeling perfectly well, but the next stage is to be seen by one of the doctors, and being examined in bed is more convenient. The Houseman will usually be the first doctor to see the patient and he will take a detailed history covering many points which may seem entirely irrelevant. However, this gives a basic profile of the patient which it may be useful to refer back to. The Houseman will then carry out a physical examination; again this will be an examination of the whole body, which may seem to have little to do with the patient's specific complaint, but it is important to have a base line from which to work and it is just as important to know and to have it recorded that bodily functions are behaving normally as it is to know about what is wrong. The Houseman may be followed by a Medical Student in some hospitals, who will duplicate his history-taking and examination.

Other doctors will also come and ask various questions and do examinations, such as the Consultant or Registrar who is going to operate, or the Anaesthetist to check the heart and lungs. It may seem that there is a lot of duplication and that communication between the doctors is poor, but doctors are taught to be suspicious of anything they are told second-hand, and they like to ask questions direct to the patient and do their own examinations. Questions asked in different ways sometimes elicit different answers which may be illuminating, and examinations carried out personally have much more meaning and impact than a second-hand account.

The nursing staff will start recording pulse rates and temperatures, which are entered on a chart, often kept at the foot of the bed. Again this is to establish what is normal for the patient as it is departures from the normal, and whether the pulse and temperature are tending to go up and down, that are significant rather than the value of an isolated reading. Blood for various tests in the laboratory may be taken. This is usually taken from a vein in the arm and is not painful; sometimes only a small quantity is required from a prick in the ear lobe or finger. Urine is also routinely examined for substances such as sugar and albumin, which should not be present in health. More complex tests such as X-rays are usually carried out in separate departments of the hospital, and the patient is taken to them, but if he is very ill it may be necessary to bring portable equipment to the bedside.

It will be found that the hospital beds are rather higher than normal beds at home. This is to make life easier for the staff, so that they are not constantly bending when making beds, etc. Usually it is possible to listen to the radio with a set of headphones which plug in near the head of the bed. There will probably be a bell-push to summon attention. In the more modern hospitals there are a selection of other facilities available at the head of the bed, such as piped oxygen and a sucker attachment for use in clinical procedures. A bed table straddles the bed, from which to eat, and for general convenience, and there will be a bedside locker for personal possessions.

Old wards are usually open with a line of beds down each side and curtains or screens to pull between the beds. The modern trend is for smaller units of one- to eight-bedded rooms, grouped into a ward. The old wards did not afford much privacy but the nursing staff were able to see at a glance the state of any patient. The modern wards are quieter and a bit less like life in a boarding school.

The mixture of apprehension, strange surroundings and the slight bustle which is inevitable, combine to hinder even people who usually have no difficulty in sleeping, from getting a good night's rest so, on settling the ward down for the night, sedatives are usually offered. These will not be obligatory except in special circumstances. A very low level of lighting will be maintained throughout the night, enabling the Night Nurse to supervise the ward without turning lights on and off, which would be more disturbing.

When an anaesthetic is to be given, it is important that the stomach is empty, to cut down the risk of vomit being inhaled into the lungs. The rule of thumb is that nothing should be given by mouth for four to six hours prior to the anaesthetic, so patients who are scheduled for operations in the morning are starved from the night before. Patients who are late on the morning list will get an early morning cup of tea, and those for the afternoon list can have a light breakfast. Before being taken to the operating theatre an injection is given which has a calming effect and also makes the mouth dry since it is much better to give an anaesthetic to a person who is not agitated, also if saliva is reduced as well as secretions in the stomach, the danger of vomiting and choking is reduced. The patient is then helped on to a trolley and taken to the theatre. He will there meet the anaesthetist in a small room adjacent to the theatre for induction of the anaesthetic. Great care will have been taken to ensure that the patient's name is clearly marked on him, usually by a piece of tape on the wrist or ankle, and that the site of the operation is clearly indicated if it is to be on a part of the body on one side or the other. At this stage a double check is made by the anaesthetist or the surgeon to ensure that the right patient is getting the right operation.

The anaesthetic is usually given by a needle into a vein in the arm, and the induction stage is very quick. The next thing that will be known is waking up, probably back in the ward. For serious operations patients are taken to a special recovery room where extra staff are available. On coming round it will often be found that there is a tube into a vein and fluid running into it, and often after an abdominal operation a tube will have been passed via the nose to the stomach. These may remain in place for a day or so, until the stomach has a chance to recover.

In the days following operations every effort will be made to get the patient mobile quickly. The days of long weeks of rest after operations have passed. Mobility helps to prevent post-operative complications such as chest infections, and the longer a patient lies in bed, the harder it will be to get him back on his feet. The physiotherapist will visit the wards and ensure that the muscle function is maintained. People who stay in hospital for a long time also find the time hanging heavily on their hands and the occupational therapist will have the job of mitigating this.

The wards are visited by many people during the course of the day, the most impressive usually being the Consultant with a retinue of Registrars, Houseman, the Sister, and other hangers on. Each patient's condition is discussed and new treatment and investigations initiated. The higher-ranking nursing officers also visit the ward periodically in a supervisory capacity. Many facilities will be brought to the patient, for instance newspapers are sold in the morning, post distributed and a library trolley will come from time to time. Telephoning can usually be done from a near-by phone if the patient is up and about, or in some hospitals a telephone trolley is brought round which can plug into a wall socket.

Hospitals vary in their attitude to visitors, the small-bedded rooms make visiting less disturbing, and often unlimited visiting is allowed, but in the old open wards fixed hours usually have to be set as a continuous stream of visitors would disrupt the ward's work too much. There is often a limit of two visitors at any one time. It is easier to allow children into small wards although they may be restricted from the big wards.

Getting information about patients' conditions can sometimes be frustrating. Phrases like "quite comfortable" and "as well as can be expected" are used frequently. This is not because medical personnel are being secretive, but because conditions change rapidly and the unexpected is always happening. Doctors and nurses find that predictions so often have a habit of being incorrect and like to stick to the present condition of a patient. If detailed information is sought, it is as well to make an appointment to see one of the doctors. He may be in the ward at the time of visiting, but he may equally well be occupied elsewhere and unavailable.

As the patients get up and about, the staff will be grateful for help in taking the tea round and in small jobs of a similar nature. It helps to pass the time, and also makes for a friendly atmosphere. Eventually the time will come for discharge, and notice is often given without much warning.

When leaving for home, a word of thanks to the ward staff is much appreciated.

23

# *Better health for parents*

Active parents are, perhaps, the most medically neglected group of people. Whatever energies they have left after looking after their own particular brood are often taken up by their own ageing parents. Mothers. perhaps, more than fathers are the chief sufferers, because the looking after of even the best-behaved single child is a round-the-clock, completely occupying, exhausting job. If there is more than one child and they are not so well behaved, the job is even more exhausting. Father does at least get out to work.

Mothers give physically. A breast-feeding mother, for example, gives part of herself to her child. It has been found in primitive areas, where nutrition is poor and children are breast-fed for two or three years, that the consistency of breast milk alters very little. This shows that if the mother's food intake is insufficient, the consistency of the milk will be maintained at her expense, and she will be physically deprived while her baby flourishes.

Of course, for the normal mother on a well-balanced diet, supplemented with the cheap milk and vitamins, breast-feeding is not detrimental to her health.

### *Balanced outlook*

What parents must realise is that if they don't look after themselves, nobody else will. Leading a normal healthy life requires certain basic ingredients like adequate food, shelter, rest, normal functioning organs and, perhaps what is most important, a balanced outlook.

How can one set about this? The first thing is to be determined that your children are neither going to overwhelm you nor split you up. The dangers are that your children will occupy you so much that you will not pursue any interests of your own. Or, more dangerous, that mother will be so occupied with the family that there will be no time left for father, and this will mean that father may tend to drift off and find all his interests and pursuits outside the home.

Try as hard as you can, however much the children swamp you, to get out on your own with your husband once a week. Better still, try to get away for a week-end together occasionally.

For general health, routine facilities offered, like mass X-ray and cervical smear tests, should be taken advantage of because they are very valuable in spotting some diseases that can be treated before they become problems. In broad lines, the time to take notice of yourself is when there is some upset or change in the normal pattern of events in your bodily function; a change in bowel habit, or an upset in the menstrual cycle; excessive weight gain or loss; increased breathlessness on effort; an unusual vaginal discharge. These should take you to your doctor.

*Watching weight*

There are certain precautions you can take. A slim person, for example, has many advantages over a fat one. Being overweight can be dangerous, and this is recognised by life insurance companies who charge you higher premiums if your weight is above the scale for your height and age. The main enemies of weight losers are carbohydrates, and a sensible intake of these is usually enough to control your weight without dieting. If, on the other hand, you are taking in less food than your body requires you are bound to lose weight, and will not gain the necessary amount unless you are taking in more food than you actually require.

Keeping slim reduces your chances of developing several troublesome conditions. These include high blood pressure, sugar diabetes, varicose veins, gall stones, toxaemia of pregnancy and fat infiltration of the heart muscles. Also, should any surgical treatment be required, a slim person is a much easier person to operate on than a fat one; and a thin agile mother is more likely to have an easier confinement than a fat one.

Unless you are grossly overweight, strict diets are not necessary. You can eat sensibly on the following basis: avoid foods like biscuits, cereals, food made with flour, sugar, sweets, chocolates, ice-cream, jams and jellies; restrict foods like bread, potatoes, fats, milk. Lean meat, game, poultry, rabbit, fish boiled or steamed, eggs in any form except fried, vegetables or fruit can be eaten freely.

The above is just a general outline of a desirable diet and it should not be difficult to follow.

Rest is important to everyone. If your children wake up continuously during the night, don't accept this as inevitable, take what steps you can by either changing routine or, if you fail in this, getting and following medical advice on the problem.

During troubled times like teething, when there is often a lot of disturbed sleep, both parents should share the load. It should be possible to arrange for each one to have at least a good night's sleep on alternate nights. No sleeping problem in children is insurmountable; they can all be solved with patience, kindness and medical help.

It is difficult to advise parents of young families what exercise to take, because in the very fact of rearing a family they are exercising themselves fairly vigorously physically. But if they are able to take up other physical games—tennis, swimming, or going for walks—these will certainly be beneficial.

Remember children grow up eventually and go their own ways. If you have spent all their childhood years giving your life completely to them, you will be left not only minus any interests of your own, but will probably leave your children with the problem of how to entertain you.

## 24

# *How to manage the family without using drugs*

The very best defence we have for illness is our own body's defence mechanism. It is amazing the number of things it can do. It can organise armies of white blood cells to repel invading germs; it can make antibodies in the blood stream that act in the same way as a poison would on other types of germs (the basis of vaccination and immunisation); it can raise the body temperature that makes other germs less active; it can cause the blood to clot when a blood vessel has been broken, sealing off the leak.

I never cease to wonder how new skin is formed after cuts and abrasions. Also in the body there are our endocrine (ductless) glands that play a part in the resistance against infection.

The first step in keeping well is to keep our defence mechanism at its absolute peak. This is achieved by generally taking care of our health and our bodies. To enable this to be effective, we have to follow some simple rules.

1. *Diet.* Diet is dealt with too frequently to go into detail, but a well-balanced diet contains a complete range of required proteins, carbohydrates, fats, vitamins, etc., providing the raw material to keep our defence mechanism in trim.

If your child's main food source is chips and bars of chocolate, and his main occupation is watching television, he is less likely to fare as well as the child who is made to eat up his vegetables, who cannot wait to get out on the football field, and who pinches an apple when given an opportunity.

2. *Exercise.* Adequate exercise is essential to keep our muscles in good tone, our chest fully expanded, and general body tissue in good vigorous shape. Starting now with a fit, healthy body, with everything working, we look for additional weapons we can add to our defence armoury.

Taking exercise, walking, organised games, gymnastics, increase the depth of our respiration, make us sweat freely, clear some of the dusty cobwebs out of our body and help us considerably in our regular bowel habit.

3. *Hygiene.* Adequate care must be taken of our outer covering of skin, keeping it clean, especially in the nooks and crannies, preventing it breaking down and cracking and presenting sites for infection. I would include in this section the care of our teeth, which must be maintained for their own sake as too easily they can become a source of infection, and for their use as mechanical food breakers. We cannot get the full advantages from our food unless it is sufficiently masticated.

Regular washing and bathing, with vigorous towelling afterwards, and a search for the points of entry of infection, like the cleft between the toes, fingernails and ears, keep the defences in a good state of order.

4. *Rest.* To recharge your batteries you must give them adequate rest, and for children this means a minimum of eight to twelve hours, with adults managing with six to eight hours, and probably even less for the elderly as they tend to take rests and catnaps during the day.

It is much more beneficial to rest in a clean, aerated room than some stuffy bunkhole where you are sharing your bed with germs, inviting them to creep in when your sentries are not looking. It is important that places of rest, and particularly bed linen, should be kept clean and well aerated.

5. *Clothing.* Clothing is necessary to protect our body from extreme ranges of temperature. It keeps the cold and wet out and prevents heat loss from our bodies. If boys are allowed to stay in their wet football shirts or go to school in wet clothes it

could cause excessive heat loss and weaken the general defence system.

Make sure in cold weather that clothing is adequate and warm, in the hot weather that it is light and loose fitting. With babies particularly, do not overdress or have too many bedclothes on. So often I am called to a restless, screaming baby with a rash, the cure for which is to remove two blankets and about six layers of clothing.

6. *Immunisation.* Take the full immunisation programme that is available. It offers protection against whooping cough, diphtheria, tetanus, polio, measles, smallpox and German measles.

* * *

It does look, so far, as if I haven't said anything at all. You were wanting advice on how to cope with your children and family when they are off colour without having to resort to drugs. All you have had so far is a keep fit regime; in fact this is the very basis of medical practice.

**IF YOU ARE TRYING TO AVOID HAVING TO USE DRUGS, TRY TO PREVENT SITUATIONS ARISING WHERE DRUGS ARE REQUIRED.**

In spite of all the precautions you have taken there will be some times when your children are off colour, off their food, etc., when they are fighting a battle against some invading force of germs or some chemical disturbance of bodily function. It is in these situations that there is a temptation to rush off for some instant remedy. But don't.

First of all take some time to enquire as to exactly what your child is complaining of. Headache, stomach ache, could be his way of saying that he is overtired and doesn't want to do something like go to school. Have a little chat together and find out exactly what is wrong. One of the best medicines is your time, your comfort, and your reassurance, and all the treatment that is required for many children's complaints is your attention. It is too easy to dish out an aspirin to see if that settles the problem, and if in fact it is a stomach ache and there is a stomach upset, rather than settle it, the aspirin could seriously aggravate it. So many upsets which we all have from time to time could be resolved simply by bed rest and taking water. This is so simple and so effective that it is too rarely tried.

*Treatment* After your chat, from what you have learnt, make a decision as to what action you are going to take. So often, in young children, over-tiredness is a large factor of whatever they are complaining of, and rest in bed will make it clear whether any further action is required.

(a) *Stomach ache and stomach upsets* Rest and water can be so effective in settling upset tummies. One of the best remedies for indigestion, both in prevention and cure, is not to rush off and buy indigestion tablets, but to rest after you have taken food rather than getting up and rushing about with a stomach full of sausage and chips, whilst your poor alimentary system is trying to digest it.

This situation is perhaps most clearly demonstrated in swimmers' cramp, which can arise by bathing too soon after a meal, the blood in your body having to split its duties in trying to take away the food supplies for storage that have been placed in the stomach and at the same time providing fuel to power the muscles and take away the waste products of muscle activity.

(b) *Coughs and colds* For coughs and colds the most important part of the treatment is to keep your children in a room of constant temperature and adequate ventilation. Too dry and too warm a room will cause the formation of sticky mucus, and it is not a cough medicine that is required but better ventilation and probably an inhalation of steam: playing Indians with your children by breathing over a bowl full of boiling water with a towel over your heads. Steam is still the most effective initial treatment in the relieving of croup.

For any illness isolation in a cold bedroom does not help, and the modern sick-room is much more likely to be a bed or a couch in front of the television set where children and adults are involved in what is going on in the rest of the house and less likely to get bored.

(c) *Bowels* Laxatives, although sometimes essential, can be disastrous and cause dehydration as well as pain and distress; you should aim to control your diet by your food intake. In babies this might mean increasing the sugar content, and in older children and adults, an increase of fruit and vegetables and bran-type foods plus an adequate fluid intake.

Most children will have got better using the simple remedies described as we recover from most things with the help only of our own defence mechanism. Some will require more treatment and advice, and the mother will then be armed with the information she has obtained from her child and her own observations of his progress. This is invaluable help if she does seek medical advice as she is able to give a full picture of what has been wrong.

The dangers of some preparations are not fully appreciated, the simple aspirin being much more dangerous than the controversial birth pill; not only can it cause ulceration and bleeding from the stomach but, when absorbed, causes some changes in our bleeding and clotting time; in over-dosage of course it is a common cause of death, and unless given under supervision and with control its very useful properties (of which there are many) are overtaken by its disadvantages.

If you manage to keep drugs out of your house you are also keeping one potential hazard away. An increasing number of conditions arise from tablet poisoning. Children getting hold of tablets that are left carelessly around, adults repeating doses of tablets, not remembering whether they have taken them or not. If there are no tablets, nobody can take any.

You keep your family fit without using drugs by ensuring that they are in the best physical health to resist illness. You take time to really find out what they are complaining of when they feel unwell. You then try the remedies of care, rest and attention, which is enough for so many conditions and is perhaps more often called "a bit of love".

If we have a serious illness or infection and our own defence mechanism does not look as if it is going to cope on its own, we are able to call in skilled help in the way of doctors and prescribed medicines. They are called to our aid when certain kinds of infection appear. Taking two examples—pneumonia and appendicitis—although it is sometimes possible in both these conditions for our body's defences to cope with the situation, it is such a long, stormy battle, with uncertainty about the end result, that we call in antibiotics to resolve the pneumonia, and surgeons to remove the appendix, two tried remedies that change these from potential grave illnesses to comparatively minor ones. This is excellent and one of the measures of how far man has become proficient in keeping his body in good repair.

We have got so used to magic cures for this type of major illness that there is the natural tendency to fly off and buy magic remedies for all the trivial minor ailments that are part of normal life and health. Few families do not have some sort of stock of proprietary remedies, supplemented by rushing to the chemist's at the first sign of minor symptoms. Too often children with colds are assaulted by their parents with aspirins, nasal drops, cough medicines, laxatives, or chest vaporising ointments, when all the real treatment required is a bowl of hot soup and a good supply of paper handkerchiefs.

The total cost of drugs on the National Health Service is enormous. Part of this is through some individual items being very expensive, but the total number of items is vast. In spite of all the medicines being prescribed, there is at least double the amount being bought over the counter, unprescribed. There is some safeguard if these preparations are bought at a chemist's as there is always a pharmacist on duty to give advice or suggest referral to a doctor. But many preparations can be bought freely in supermarkets with no accompanying available advice. But mothers who have read this book will not be amongst the purchasers either at chemists or supermarkets as they know how to keep their family fit without using drugs.

# Index